SOLVING PATI

Inte

Medicine

Solving Patient Problems:

Internal Medicine

William J. Mitchell, M.D.

Clinical Associate Professor
Department of Medicine
University of New Mexico School of Medicine
Director of Physician Resources
Catholic Health Initiatives
Albuquerque, New Mexico

Steve M. Mitchell, M.D.

Senior Research Scientist
Director of Computers in Medical Education
University of New Mexico School of Medicine
Albuquerque, New Mexico

Typesetter: Pagesetters, Brattleboro, VT
Printer: Port City Press, Baltimore, MD

Distributors:

United States and Canada
Blackwell Science, Inc.
Commerce Place
350 Main Street
Malden, MA 02148
Telephone orders: 800-215-1000 or 781-388-8250
Fax orders: 781-388-8270

Australia
Blackwell Science, PTY LTD.
54 University Street
Carlton, Victoria 3053
Telephone orders: 61-39-347-0300
Fax orders: 61-39-347-5001

Outside North America and Australia
Blackwell Science, LTD.
c/o Marston Book Service, LTD.
P.O. Box 269
Abingdon Oxon, OX 14 4XN England
Telephone orders: 44-1-235-465500
Fax orders: 44-1-235-465555

2 3 4 5 6 7 8 9 10

Contents

Preface

Erasmus, who lived during the late 15th and early 16th centuries, is said to be the last human being who was capable of knowing all of the knowledge acquired in history. As with the entire fund of human knowledge, the science of medicine is growing exponentially.

I remember when I was a second-year medical student and struggling to memorize all of the different adrenoreceptors, I angrily asked my father how he tackled this seemingly unending task when he was in medical school. To my surprise, he answered, "I didn't. When I was in medical school, no one knew anything about adrenoreceptors or any other receptor for that matter!" Just two decades ago, the medical database did not yet include what is now one of the fundamental principles of physiology. It appears that the known sum of medical knowledge is perhaps growing too large for any individual to grasp.

Clearly, the body of medical knowledge will continue to grow, leaving us a couple of choices: extend medical school beyond 4 years (not a financially or emotionally palatable solution) or change the approach to learning medicine.

In a way, medicine is traditionally taught backwards; that is, students are first taught normal physiology, then pathophysiology, and then are introduced to the symptoms that may result in disease. Unfortunately, patients present first with symptoms, which requires physicians to work backwards to figure out the pathophysiology.

This text presents a problem-based approach to learning medicine, which is the same way that physicians actually practice medicine: from symptom to diagnosis rather than the more traditional diagnosis to symptom. In doing so, we hope to at least attempt a partial solution to the "knowledge explosion" problem. Since we cannot hope to know everything, we might instead learn the basic principles of medicine and then apply these principles to clinical problem-solving. Rather than presenting long lists of diagnoses for memorization, we present common clinical complaints (symptoms) and guide you through the problem-solving process. We hope to introduce you to patient presentations that are common in internal medicine, thereby giving you the means with which to address a wide range of patient complaints. Obviously we cannot present all of the diagnoses that you will encounter during your medical student years. However, we hope to give you the tools with which to solve many patient problems. In addition, we hope to offer you a means of learning medicine that is more interesting and more exciting than rote memorization.

STEVE M. MITCHELL, M.D.

To our wives, Eleanor and Wendy, for putting up with us while we labored in this endeavor.

To Osa, for always being there.

Introduction

One of the major problems in medical education is that the traditional approach (memory-based approach) to educating future physicians inadequately prepares them for clinical problem-solving. Thus, problem-based learning was designed to place the teaching of content (and memorization) and problem-solving skills on an equal footing. Surveys of both traditional and problem-based educational programs have determined the following: most students in traditional programs feel that more than 50% of what they learn is memorized without understanding; however, most students in problem-based programs feel that less than 20% of what they learn is memorized without understanding. Unfortunately, because of the deficiencies in the traditional (memory-based) approach to medicine, students are handicapped by their memorization of large amounts of information that they are unable to apply to clinical problems.

These books are designed to help the reader develop an approach to clinical problem-solving. While traditional medical education demands that students memorize vast amounts of information without understanding, problem-based learning is based on the concept of practicing the process of problem-solving while acquiring the knowledge (content) used in the process. George Bordage, M.D.,[1] states in his article "Elaborated Knowledge" that "less is better for beginning students when introducing new material"; that is, in order for the student to be able to organize information for later recall, less information, preferably using prototypical case presentations, must be provided so that students are able to understand, incorporate, and then use what they learn. Students who have the most trouble with clinical reasoning seem to have a poorly organized knowledge base, making rational approaches to patient problems almost impossible.

There is no question that knowledge is important in problem-solving. The more the student knows, the better he or she can test the hypotheses that are entertained. It is the quality of the hypotheses and the skill in testing them that distinguish the expert from the novice. Failure to consider more than one hypotheses is one of the basic deficiences of inexperience. One of the goals of this text is

[1] Bordage G: Elaborated knowledge: a key to successful diagnostic thinking. *Acad Med* 69:883–885, 1994. George Bordage, M.D., is Professor and Director of Graduate Studies in the Department of Medical Education at the College of Medicine, University of Illinois at Chicago, Chicago, Illinois.

to help the student move from novice to expert in this critical area of medical diagnosis.

The purpose of the *Solving Patient Problems Series* is to assist students at all levels in developing their clinical problem-solving or reasoning skills by leading them through the clinical reasoning process around common presenting complaints in the various clinical rotations. The most common diseases that students are likely to encounter given the chief complaints are presented. These prototypical diseases are the foundation upon which students may then begin to build a more extensive differential. Only by comparing and contrasting the diagnostic features of two or more common diseases can students build a knowledge base that will allow the inclusion of other possible causes of the same complaint, thereby moving from prototypical problems to more complex problems and then to life-threatening problems that must not be overlooked.

The chapters are organized around common presenting complaints. A patient case is presented, followed by questions concerning additional data that may be needed. The questions are then followed by a discussion that answers the questions raised previously. A physical examination and laboratory studies are presented next, followed by another series of questions that should lead the student either closer to the diagnosis or to the diagnosis. An assessment, including the differential and a resolution, follow. Chapters organized in this way can be used for study, learning, assessment, and review. The presentations followed by questions allow students to do their own reasoning before reading the authors' discussions. Sidebars provide the "pearls" from each case but can also serve as reminders of important facts when reviewing.

In no way is this text meant to be inclusive but rather a supplement, guide, and aid to the success of students as diagnosticians. It is deliberately pocket-sized to be carried on clinical rotations. More extensive reading about patients is necessary. However, facts learned about diseases in the context of patient presentations are bound to be easier to retain and retrieve. What seems to be "intuition" and part of the "art" of medicine is actually a combination of experience and a very highly organized knowledge base, which allows physicians to differentiate quickly between differential diagnoses—a necessary skill that this text has been designed to help students develop.

S. SCOTT OBENSHAIN, M.D.[2]

---

[2]S. Scott Obenshain, M.D., is the Associate Dean for Undergraduate Medical Education and Professor of Pediatrics and Family and Community Medicine at the University of New Mexico School of Medicine, Albuquerque, New Mexico.

CHAPTER 1
Chief Complaint:
Unintentional Weight Loss

CASE 1-1

INITIAL PRESENTATION

Mrs. G. is a 52-year-old Hispanic office manager who presents to a clinic with the complaint of fatigue and weight loss. Mrs. G. states that she first began feeling unusually "worn out" at the end of the day roughly 4 months ago. Since that time, her energy level has been gradually decreasing. Currently, she is concerned because she is having difficulty working throughout the day and is worried that her job is in jeopardy. Upon further questioning, Mrs. G. explained that she has "no energy" but does not feel sleepy. Her sleeping patterns have not changed except that within the last several months she has been getting up several times a night to urinate. She can usually get back to sleep easily and is not concerned by this. She can think of no reason why she might feel fatigued. Mrs. G. also notes a 10-lb weight loss during the past 4 months. She states that she has "always had trouble keeping her weight down," and she tries to walk regularly. Mrs. G. thinks this weight loss is peculiar because she has not been able to walk as far or as often as she used to because of her lack of energy. She stated that she always tries to eat three "healthy" meals a day and that her appetite has not changed. Mrs. G. has no other symptoms of which she is aware, including no changes in bowel habits. Her medical history is significant for hypothyroidism, and she has been on a stable dose of L-thyroxine. For 10 years she has also taken lovastatin for elevated cholesterol and lisinopril for hypertension. Mrs. G. is postmenopausal and on hormone replacement therapy (HRT). Her father has "heart problems," and her mother died of "some kind of cancer" at age 62. Her family history is otherwise unremarkable.

> Weight loss with progressively worsening fatigue

> No change in diet

> Significant medical and family histories

1. What further questions should the physician ask the patient?
2. What aspects of Mrs. G.'s family history require more questioning?

Discussion

Further questioning and a chart review reveal the following pieces of information. Mrs. G. was diagnosed with hypothyroidism 10 years ago, after she noted weight gain, fatigue, and cold intolerance. She currently exhibits none of these symptoms; however, her thyroid hormone levels have not been checked in more than 1 year. Her elevated cholesterol level was diagnosed 14 years ago, and her records indicate that it has been well controlled on her current therapy. Her hypertension was diagnosed 7 years ago and has also been well controlled. Further questioning reveals that Mrs. G.'s

> **No history of heart disease**

father has had heart problems since he was a child, but Mrs. G. cannot be more specific. She denies chest pain, palpitations, diaphoresis, lightheadedness, and shortness of breath. She also denies cough, fever, chills, sweats, exposure to infectious diseases, or risk factors for human immunodeficiency virus. A review of old records indicates that the patient's mother died of pancreatic cancer. She is postmenopausal and has been on HRT for several years but has recently been having trouble with intermittent spotting. She reports that she is seeing her gynecologist for this problem. Mrs. G. notes no recent change in her moods and describes her emotional state as "generally very happy." When asked about increased thirst, Mrs. G. reports that she drinks water constantly throughout the day. She also urinates frequently, including three or four times during the night.

3. What possible conditions can be considered initially to explain this patient's weight loss?

As with any condition, the associated symptoms and other medical history may provide important diagnostic clues. In this case, fatigue may be helpful, although it is often nonspecific. Fatigue associated with thyroid disease usually indicates hypothyroidism, and thus weight gain rather than weight loss would be expected if her thyroid hormone replacement therapy were inadequate. Excessive thyroid hormone replacement causes a hypermetabolic state, which may result in hyperactivity, but fatigue is often prominent. Furthermore, weight loss usually occurs in this situation. Virtually any chronic illness may manifest as weight loss. Heart disease, for example, can present with weight loss unless there is significant fluid retention. This patient has hypertension, high cholesterol, and a family history of "heart problems," all of which may be risk factors for coronary artery disease. Of course, cancer may present as weight loss, so further inquiry into Mrs. G.'s mother's illness would be warranted. Diabetes often presents with weight loss and fatigue, as does anemia. Lastly, fatigue and weight changes are both common symptoms of clinical depression.

4. What should the physician look for during the physical examination?
5. What laboratory tests may help differentiate the cause of Mrs. G.'s condition?

PHYSICAL EXAMINATION

During the physical examination, Mrs. G. was noted to be 5'4" and 144 lbs, with a temperature of 99°F, a pulse of 88 beats/min, and blood pressure of 136/80 mm Hg. The physician noted her general appearance as such: "Mrs. G. is a moderately overweight female in no apparent distress. She is friendly and smiles frequently." Mucous membranes were noted to be without pallor. Her skin was described as being of normal texture; lesions or rashes were not noted. Her cardiac and pulmonary examinations showed no abnormalities. All of her reflexes exhibited a normal relaxation time, and the rest of her physical examination was unremarkable.

LABORATORY TESTS

The laboratory tests performed were noninvasive and relatively inexpensive, yet they provided significant information pertaining to Mrs. G.'s possible problems. The results of these tests were:

Laboratory Tests	Patient	Normal Values
White blood cell (WBC) count	6200/mL	4800–10,500/mL
Thyroid-stimulating hormone (TSH)	3 mIU/L	0.5–6 mIU/L
Hemoglobin	12 g/dL	12–16 g/dL
Hematocrit	38%	37%–47%
Hemoglobin A_{1c} (HbA_{1c})	9.8%	4.0%–7.0%

6. How does the information from the physical examination help in differentiating the possible causes?
7. How do laboratory results affect the differential diagnosis?
8. How has the differential diagnosis evolved?

9. Are there any other laboratory tests that could have been performed? What results would be expected?
10. What is the final diagnosis in this case?

Discussion

The TSH level is normal, indicating that Mrs. G.'s thyroid hormone replacement medication is adequate. Her decreased hemoglobin level and hematocrit are likely due, in part, to her history of vaginal bleeding, but the cause should be explored. As noted in the initial presentation, Mrs. G. is currently being evaluated by her gynecologist. Although the hemoglobin level and hematocrit are on the low end of "normal," they are not low enough to explain fully her current symptoms. There are no signs or symptoms of chronic infectious diseases such as tuberculosis or osteomyelitis. There is nothing to suggest collagen diseases such as lupus erythematosus or rheumatoid arthritis.

ASSESSMENT

Given her elevated HbA_{1c}, **type 2 diabetes mellitus (type 2 DM)** is the most likely cause for both fatigue and weight loss. In fact, Mrs. G.'s presentation is fairly typical for this disorder. Mrs. G. is slightly overweight, which decreases insulin sensitivity. This is a risk factor for type 2 DM, which has an insidious onset similar to what Mrs. G. is experiencing. She presents with both fatigue and weight loss because diabetes is essentially a state of starvation. Glucose levels are too high in her blood because sugar cannot be transported intracellularly. In effect, the intracellular environment is "starved" for sugar. As a result, the body switches to a catabolic state. Fats are broken down as an alternative energy source, which explains Mrs. G.'s weight loss. Also, the patient's history of hypothyroidism may be significant in that hypothyroidism frequently occurs with diabetes, possibly because of a common underlying autoimmune pathology.

11. What are the basic mechanisms of weight loss?

Discussion

Weight loss is not an uncommon problem in internal medicine, and the diagnosis is often elusive. However, the patient's history, along with a basic understanding of fat, carbohydrate, and protein metabolism, can be very helpful. In trying to understand the various aspects of metabolism, it is useful to think of two basic states: fasting and fed. In the fasting state, the body depends on endogenous substrates for energy generation. Insulin levels are low, so glucose is not taken up by peripheral tissues and is spared for use by the central nervous system (CNS). In adipose tissue, triglycerides are hydrolyzed to free fatty acids (FFAs), which are then oxidized by muscle tissue. The liver also oxidizes FFAs to produce ketoacids, acetoacetate, and β-hydroxybutyrate, which can be used as oxidative substrates by the muscles and CNS. Proteins are catabolized into amino acids, which can be used by the liver for gluconeogenesis. The overall result is a switch in substrate use by peripheral tissues to spare glucose for oxidation by the CNS. Unlike most peripheral tissues, the brain does not require insulin for intracellular transport of glucose. Thus, when fuel is low, the brain is spared at the expense of other tissues.

For practical purposes, the fed state is exactly the reverse. In this case, both glucose and other substrates abound, and anabolic processes predominate. Insulin levels are high, which allow glucose to be stored in liver and muscle as glycogen or converted to triglycerides for storage in adipose tissue. Ingested fats are also stored as triglycerides in adipose tissue, and amino acids are synthesized into protein. In the fed state, fatty acid oxidation and ketogenesis are greatly decreased. In very basic terms, factors that create a fasting state inevitably cause eventual weight loss. Mrs. G. reports no change in eating or exercise habits, which may indicate that a pathologic process is occurring.

In general, weight loss can be divided into two categories: increased food intake and decreased food intake. The former includes such etiologies as thyrotoxicosis, diabetes, and malabsorption diseases. The latter category suggests neoplasia or chronic failure of lungs, heart, kidneys, or liver, as well as mood disorders and diseases such as gastric ulcers, in which symptoms may worsen with food intake. Chronic multisystem disorders, such as collagen vascular diseases and infectious processes with slow progression, may also cause weight loss but the mechanisms are less clear.

Mrs. G. returns to the clinic 3 months after being placed on the American Diabetes Association diet and an oral antidiabetic agent (i.e., glyburide). She is now concerned about a 10-lb weight gain during this period of time. Mrs. G., however, reports feeling "much better." Her excessive thirst and urination have resolved, and her energy has returned. A physical examination indicates a documented 9-lb weight gain in the past 3 months. Laboratory testing shows her HbA_{1c} level to be 6.5%; improved from 9.8%.

12. What is the diagnosis for Mrs. G. at this point?
13. What action should the physician recommend?

This is the exact reverse of what was happening to Mrs. G. when she first presented to the clinic. When her diabetes began, she was in a fasting state, and her cells were literally starved for nutrients. Once the diabetes was controlled and her cells were "fed" again, her metabolism changed to an anabolic state. The physician encouraged Mrs. G. to lose weight because weight gain can increase her insulin resistance and cause her glucose control to deteriorate. Together, they agreed on a diet and exercise program to decrease her weight and improve her circulation.

CASE 1-2

INITIAL PRESENTATION

A 32-year-old woman has lost 22 lbs during the past 6 months without intentionally trying to do so. The woman has experienced increasing anxiety during the same time period, as well as frequent episodes of heart "palpitations." Her other complaints include muscle weakness, loss of sleep, heat intolerance, and perhaps surprisingly, increased appetite.

PHYSICAL EXAMINATION

The woman's blood pressure is 144/92 mm Hg, her temperature is 99.4°F, and her pulse is 96 beats/min. The physician notes lid lag, a diffusely enlarged thyroid gland, and brisk bilateral reflexes with a short relaxation time.

ASSESSMENT

This patient is similar to Mrs. G. of Case 1-1 in that both note significant weight loss. However, this patient exhibits clear signs of **thyrotoxicosis,** possibly **Graves' disease.** All of the signs and symptoms noted above are consistent with Graves' disease, and thyroid function tests should be performed. Thyrotoxicosis is an interesting cause of weight loss because it usually occurs in a state of increased appetite and food intake. Despite eating more, nutritional inadequacy is almost always present. This is primarily because of an increased basal metabolic rate induced by excess thyroid hormone. Thyrotoxicosis causes increased synthesis and degradation of protein and fat, but degradation rates are always increased disproportionately. Weight loss is due to a combination of muscle wasting and the mobilization of FFAs from adipose tissue. In addition, both serum glucose levels and insulin are often increased in patients with thyrotoxicosis, suggesting the possibility that thyroid hormone interferes with insulin action.

CASE 1-3

INITIAL PRESENTATION

A 63-year-old man with a 10-lb weight loss during the past few months has a new associated symptom of dry cough. The patient has a chronic history of shortness of breath with exertion and a 60-pack-year history of smoking.

PHYSICAL EXAMINATION

The patient is a frail-appearing man who appears older than his stated age. His lungs are clear to percussion and auscultation. The physician orders a chest radiograph, which shows a well-defined 2–3-cm rounded mass lesion in the upper right lobe.

ASSESSMENT

This case is certainly suggestive of a **chronic illness–induced weight loss.** There are no specific symptoms that can be tied directly to weight loss. However, this patient does have a significant risk history for a variety of chronic illnesses. His history of smoking and new-onset dry cough would be consistent either with a pulmonary problem or a cardiac disorder, such as congestive heart failure (CHF). CHF can occasionally cause weight loss. However, the absence of other cardiac history and pulmonary congestion on examination make this a less likely diagnosis. The chest radiograph is highly suspicious for a pulmonary neoplasm. Malignancies of any kind, but particularly those in the gastrointestinal tract, lung, or lymphatic system, can produce weight loss. Unfortunately, weight loss does not usually become significant until such neoplasms have advanced significantly. In most cases, the weight loss associated with cancer occurs secondary to diminished dietary intake, and this case differs from the patients in Case 1-1 and Case 1-2 in this respect. Like the other two patients, however, this man is in a relative fasting state.

CASE 1-4

INITIAL PRESENTATION

A 44-year-old woman complaining of a 20-lb weight loss during the past year has been seen numerous times in the clinic for various aches and pains of unknown etiology. She reports difficulty sleeping, complains of fatigue and lethargy, and is unable to hold a job. The woman lives alone and has been divorced for 2 years.

PHYSICAL EXAMINATION

The patient appears lethargic, but her physical examination is otherwise normal. There are no localized findings.

LABORATORY TESTS

Laboratory test results were as follows:

Laboratory Tests	Patient
TSH	Normal
HbA$_{1c}$	Normal
CBC	Normal

ASSESSMENT

Mood disorders such as **depression** are one of the most common causes of weight change. Depression often manifests with somatic complaints, sleep disturbances, fatigue or lethargy, and work or social difficulties. However, basic screening for endocrine or hematologic disorders is often necessary to rule out primary causes. This case, as with all of the others, is an example of a situation in which the body is in a fasting state. It is also similar to Case 1-3 in that the primary cause for weight loss is decreased food intake. She will be referred for psychiatric evaluation and possibly antidepressant medications.

CASE 1-5

INITIAL PRESENTATION

A 66-year-old man complains of a 15-lb weight gain over the past 2 months. He has had coronary artery disease for 17 years and sustained two previous heart attacks. The man reports increasing shortness of breath, particularly when supine. A slight nonproductive cough is also exacerbated by lying down.

PHYSICAL EXAMINATION

This patient's physical examination shows a normal cardiac rate with a third heart sound (S_3) gallop. In both lower extremities, 1+ pitting edema is noted. A chest radiograph shows an enlarged heart with bilateral lower lobe infiltrates.

ASSESSMENT

CHF was discussed earlier as one of many conditions that could potentially cause weight loss primarily due to decreased food intake. However, this case illustrates that CHF may also induce **weight gain secondary to fluid retention.** This patient's history of dyspnea and coronary artery disease, coupled with the physical findings of an S_3 gallop, lower extremity edema, and a chest radiograph showing an enlarged heart with bilateral infiltrates, are consistent with CHF. When cardiac output is diminished, the juxtaglomerular apparatus of the kidneys senses hypovolemia due to relative lack of perfusion. This, in turn, stimulates the renin-angiotensin–aldosterone system, eventually resulting in water and salt retention with a consequent weight gain. S_3 gallop refers to the sound of rapid, turbulent filling of the ventricles and is consistent with fluid overload. Simultaneously increased fluid volume causes an increase in hydrostatic pressure in the lower extremities resulting in edema.

Weight gain is presented here as a contrast to the previous discussions on weight loss and because it is a common complaint encountered in internal medicine. Generally, pathologic weight gain can be attributed to a continuous fed state, which may be induced by various endocrine changes such as hypothyroidism, improvement in diabetes control, or recovery from hyperthyroidism. Furthermore, as this case demonstrates, water retention caused by potentially serious diseases (e.g., heart or renal failure) can occasionally present as weight gain and, therefore, must be ruled out.

SUMMARY

Unintentional weight loss often presents a difficult diagnostic problem for a physician because many different pathologies and systems may be involved. The approach to a patient with unintentional weight loss, however, may be aided by keeping some very basic principles in mind. A careful dietary history, for example, is often crucial. In particular, it is essential to determine whether the patient's appetite has decreased or increased. Weight loss in the context of an increased appetite suggests that the body's appetite regulating system is functioning properly but that food intake is not matching energy needs either due to malabsorption, hyper-metabolism, or a dysfunction in substrate delivery to tissues. Examples include pancreatic insufficiency, hyperthyroidism, and diabetes mellitus, respectively. Weight loss in the setting of a decreased appetite, however, suggests that the body is not properly regulating its own food intake. This situation often presents much more of a diagnostic problem because the etiologies are so variable. Virtually any chronic ailment may cause a lack of appetite. In particular, chronic degenerative disorders, neoplasia, or mood disorders are suspect. In addition, consideration of diseases such as PUD or esophagitis, which may cause pain or discomfort with food intake may be warranted. Once it is clear whether or not a patient's appetite is increased or decreased, then an assessment of associated symptoms and a medical history can usually further discern the most likely etiology well enough to establish which physical examination maneuvers and laboratory investigations are warranted.

CHAPTER 2
Chief Complaint: Abdominal Pain and Chills

CASE 2-1

INITIAL PRESENTATION

Mr. O. is a 44-year-old, unemployed construction worker who comes into the emergency department complaining of sharp abdominal pain and chills during the past 12 hours. Mr. O. states that he has not felt particularly well for the past 2 days but thought it was just the "flu." He awoke this morning with severe midepigastric pain. He states that within a few hours he noticed that the pain spread to his back. Mr. O. describes the pain as nonvarying and excruciating. He states that he has also been somewhat nauseated. He has no

> Localizing symptomatology

diarrhea and has not vomited. The patient has never had an illness such as this before and notes no preceding symptoms. He has no chronic illnesses and takes no medications on a regular basis. He has a 30-pack-year history of smoking and has never used any illegal drugs. Further questioning reveals that Mr. O. drinks alcohol regularly. He tells you that he is a whiskey drinker. For all of his adult life, he has imbibed three to four glasses of whiskey per day and is a binge drinker on weekends. Five months ago, he lost his job as a construction worker; he has since doubled his alcohol intake. Mr. O. blames most of his increased alcohol use on the fact that his wife moved out 4 months ago. He has never had gallbladder problems, liver disease, or ulcers as far as he knows.

> Possible risk factors

The medical history is unremarkable except for occasional upset stomach and minor abdominal pain following heavy bouts of drinking. The family history includes the fact that the patient's father was an alcoholic.

1. Does severe abdominal pain that begins acutely help narrow the diagnostic possibilities?
2. What is the significance of abdominal pain that spreads or radiates to the back?

3. What does the history of chills tell you?
4. What abdominal pathology is more likely with a history of alcohol abuse?

Discussion

Abdominal pain is a very common complaint in internal medicine. Pathology in virtually any organ in the pelvis, chest, and abdomen can cause abdominal pain. In this particular case, however, there are some significant factors in the history that help narrow the differential diagnosis. It should be noted, for example, that this patient's pain began acutely and is quite severe. As with other systems in the body, acute illnesses often suggest inflammation, infection, or other rapidly progressing pathologies such as a perforation or obstruction. In addition, this patient's history of chills would support an infectious or inflammatory process. The pain radiating to the back is also a helpful clue. In contrast to the parietal peritoneum, the visceral peritoneum has little sensory innervation. As a result, many abdominal pathologies initially present as dull, diffuse pain. However, as the process worsens, and portions of the peritoneum adherent to the abdominal wall become inflamed, the pain often becomes localized. Abdominal pain radiating to the back suggests that retroperitoneal organs (e.g., the pancreas, the duodenum, or occasionally the kidneys) may be involved. Perhaps the most significant portion of this patient's medical history is his reported alcohol intake. Alcohol abuse is a risk factor for a variety of gastrointestinal (GI) disorders such as esophagitis, peptic ulcer disease (PUD), and pancreatitis.

PHYSICAL EXAMINATION

Physical examination reveals the following: The patient's vital signs are significant for a temperature of 100°F. His blood pressure is 112/78 mm Hg, and his heart rate is 96 beats/min. The patient is sitting hunched forward on the examination table and appears to be in severe pain. A lung examination is significant for crackles in the left base with pain in this region on deep inspiration. An abdominal examination reveals a slightly distended but soft abdomen with decreased bowel sounds. There is slight voluntary guarding. The rest of the physical examination is unremarkable. The review of systems is negative except as noted in the present illness.

5. Does sitting hunched forward indicate a specific problem?
6. How might the lung findings relate to abdominal pathology?

Discussion

The physical examination confirms that this patient's pain is indeed severe, and it also conveys some information as to the location and extent of this pathology. The lack of peritoneal signs indicates that there is no peritonitis. The patient is leaning forward, possibly to alleviate pressure on retroperitoneal organs. In addition, the lung crackles and pain on deep inspiration clearly indicate pulmonary involvement. Given the localized severity of this man's pain, a reasonable assumption at this point would be that the lung involvement is probably somehow secondary to an abdominal disorder and not a primary etiology. Inflammation just under a hemidiaphragm may spread chemically across the diaphragm and result in an inflammatory process involving the pleura and base of the lung.

LABORATORY TESTS

7. What laboratory tests should be ordered for this patient?

Discussion

At this point, a primary abdominal pathology is certainly suspect. In particular, there is evidence that retroperitoneal organs are involved; therefore, laboratory tests should be directed to rule in or out those etiologies that could affect retroperitoneal organs. In addition, a chest radiograph is reasonable because of the apparent lung involvement.

A chest radiograph shows left-sided pleural effusion; a plain abdominal radiograph is normal. Liver function tests indicated mildly elevated transaminases, mildly elevated conjugated bilirubin, and an alkaline phosphatase level 1.5 times normal. Serum electrolyte levels were normal. Results of other laboratory tests were as follows:

Laboratory Tests	Patient	Normal Values
White blood cell (WBC)	14,000	5000–10,000
Serum amylase	200 cup/L	35–115 cup/L
Serum lipase	230 U/L	60–80 U/L
Serum calcium	280 U/L	0–160 U/L

8. What is the significance of an elevation in conjugated bilirubin?
9. Where are amylase and lipase made?

Lipase and amylase assays were performed on this patient because both his history of alcohol intake and signs and symptoms of retroperitoneal involvement strongly suggest acute pancreatitis as a diagnosis. Numerous conditions, including elevated triglycerides, can cause pancreatitis, but gallstones and alcohol abuse are by far the most common etiologic factors. Elevated serum amylase is the hallmark of pancreatitis. However, it should be noted that increased amylase levels may also occur in many other conditions such as salivary disease, diabetic ketoacidosis, renal insufficiency (decreased clearance), dissecting aneurysms, nonpancreatic tumors, and a variety of gynecologic and intestinal disorders. Likewise, a normal amylase level does not necessarily rule out pancreatitis because roughly one-third of these patients present with normal levels. In this case, the history coupled with the increase in amylase strongly suggests acute pancreatitis as the diagnosis. Elevation of the serum lipase level to greater than three times normal is more specific but slightly less sensitive than the amylase level and is therefore helpful to confirm the diagnosis. Pleural effusions are not uncommon in patients with acute pancreatitis. Cholecystitis may cause increased serum amylase levels as well as an associated pancreatitis. Thus, it may often be difficult to delineate these two disorders even with evidence of gallstones.

PUD is also a consideration in this patient, as it can occasionally cause increased serum amylase and lipase levels; this patient's history of alcohol abuse puts him at risk for PUD. A perforated duodenal ulcer would likely produce retroperitoneal inflammation symptoms such as pain radiating to the back, and there may be associated pancreatitis causing increased lipase levels. However, the lack of peritoneal signs and the absence of free air seen on the abdominal radiograph both tend to make this diagnosis less likely. Mesenteric vascular disease also can cause elevations in serum amylase and lipase levels and could certainly present as severe abdominal pain.

Unfortunately, as these examples illustrate, almost any acute abdominal disorder can theoretically cause transient increases in serum lipase and amylase levels and mild increases in the liver enzymes. The approach to any patient with abdominal pain, therefore, requires diligent analysis and integration of all of the signs and symptoms, often only to arrive at a presumptive diagnosis. As a result, treatment frequently consists of maintenance of normal fluid balance, pain control, and observation. In this particular case, the subjective and objective data make many of the above referenced disorders less likely. The absence of any localized right upper quadrant pain, for example, coupled with only mild elevations in liver function tests, tend to rule out hepatic or gallbladder involvement. Mesenteric vessel ischemia is a possibility in this patient given the acuteness and severity of his symptoms, although the absence of recurrent postprandial pain preceding the onset of his current symptoms makes this somewhat less likely, unless the vasculature were compromised acutely as with an embolic phenomenon. In addition, pain radiating to the back strongly indicates retroperitoneal involvement such as pancreatitis, a diagnosis that is supported by this patient's history of alcohol abuse and increased levels of serum amylase and lipase.

Although an absolutely definitive diagnosis can be made only with surgical intervention, acute pancreatitis is certainly the most likely diagnosis at this point. Mild white blood cell (WBC) elevation and pleural effusions are common in patients with acute pancreatitis. Conjugated bilirubin is elevated when the biliary tract is obstructed, as with a gallstone or with edema of the bile duct from an inflammatory process (such as pancreatitis) in the region. The absence of free air on the abdominal radiograph helps rule out an intestinal perforation, such as a perforated duodenal ulcer. Further diagnostic testing such as ultrasound, computed tomography (CT) scan, or endoscopic retrograde cholangiopancreatography (ERCP) would not be unreasonable in this case, although they may or may not yield any definitive results. Monitoring fluid balance and blood chemistries would also be extremely important in this patient because hypovolemia and hypocalcemia are common with this condition.

ASSESSMENT

Based on a presumptive diagnosis of **acute pancreatitis** the treatment plan for this patient is admittance to the hospital for fluid and electrolyte balance, pain control, and observation for complications. He has no evidence of dehydration, but this can occur through fluid losses in the retroperitoneum. Fluid replacement must be done with careful monitoring of electrolytes and appropriate replacement where indicated. Oral intake must be avoided so that pancreatic secretions are not stimulated. Meperidine may be used to control pain. Initial complications for which to look include massive fluid loss resulting in shock, severe hypocalcemia and hypomagnesemia, and adult respiratory distress syndrome. These events require monitoring in an intensive care unit. In cases of severe pancreatitis, the acute phase may last 2 weeks, and, if the patient survives, may lead to long-term complications. The most common complications involve collections of fluid and inflammatory debris in and around the pancreas. These pockets may be pseudocysts or abscesses and should be suspected if there is persistent fever, abdominal pain, or delayed recovery of normal GI function. An abdominal CT scan is necessary to define such complications further.

Most cases of acute pancreatitis resolve in less than 1 week, with appropriate treatment. Approximately 5%–25% of patients with pancreatitis have complications such as those described above. After recovery, efforts to avoid a recurrence are paramount because repeated bouts may destroy the pancreatic endocrine and exocrine functions, resulting in diabetes and pancreatic enzyme deficiencies. If gallstones are the precipitating factor, they must be removed surgically. Any hypertriglyceridemia must be treated with diet or medication. Abstinence from alcohol is essential, and, if necessary, an alcohol rehabilitation program should be encouraged.

CASE 2-2

INITIAL PRESENTATION

A 38-year-old man complains of abdominal pains during the past 2 years. He describes his pains as dull and tending to wax and wane but, in general, not getting better or worse. There are no associated abdominal or GI symptoms. As a financial consultant who has been losing many accounts in the past 2 years, he has had increasing difficulties with work and family life.

PHYSICAL EXAMINATION

The patient's general appearance is sullen and melancholy. There is no localizable abdominal discomfort on deep abdominal palpation. The remainder of the physical examination is within normal limits.

LABORATORY TESTS

Laboratory tests included electrolytes, a complete blood count (CBC), an abdominal radiograph, and liver function tests, all of which were within normal limits.

ASSESSMENT

10. Does the 2-year duration of pain with lack of symptom progression suggest serious abdominal pathology?

Discussion

Unlike Mr. O. in Case 2-1, this patient's symptoms are notably less severe and obviously more chronic. As a result, vascular, occlusive, or infectious processes are unlikely. Of further note in this case is the absence of any localizing symptoms or abnormal laboratory values. Depression very commonly presents as nondescript somatic complaints, such as abdominal pain. Unfortunately, primary depression is often a diagnosis of exclusion, and chronic illness or pain may frequently result in secondary depression. This presents the physician with the "chicken or egg" dilemma. The question is always how far to proceed with laboratory tests before assigning the diagnosis of primary depression. This patient may undergo further evaluation with CT or magnetic resonance imaging (MRI). However, if there is strong historical evidence of depression and an absence of physical or laboratory findings, primary clinical depression is always suspect.

The diagnosis of this patient is **chronic depression.** The treatment plan involves ruling out any suicidal ideation and evaluating further the need for counseling, pharmaceutical intervention, or referral to a psychiatrist.

CASE 2-3

INITIAL PRESENTATION

A 38-year-old woman presents with moderately severe, diffuse, cramping abdominal pain that woke her up 6 hours ago and is worsening in the periumbilical region. She reports associated anorexia and nausea but states that she has not traveled recently, has not had dietary changes, has no history of surgery, is not currently sexually active, and has no urinary symptoms or changes. Her last menstrual period was 2 weeks ago.

PHYSICAL EXAMINATION

The woman's temperature is 100°F. There are no masses in her abdomen, but there is diffuse tenderness to palpation with voluntary guarding, as well as a positive psoas sign. The remainder of the physical examination is within normal limits.

ASSESSMENT

Like the case of Mr. O., this patient has acute-onset abdominal pain. In general, acute onset tends to indicate a vascular, infectious, or obstructive problem. The "cramping" nature of the pain suggests spasms. The diffuse pain, as in the first case, may indicate that the peritoneum is (as yet) not involved. The associated symptoms of nausea and anorexia are difficult to interpret because many disorders eventually manifest as such. As with the case of Mr. O., there are literally hundreds of possibilities that might explain these signs and symptoms. However, as discussed earlier, the acute nature helps to limit the possibilities. Although mesenteric artery ischemia is a consideration, it is unlikely in a young, otherwise healthy adult, especially with no preceding symptoms. It is also important to keep in mind other organs in the abdomen besides the GI tract. Disorders of the genitourinary system, for example, often present with abdominal pain. For a woman in her reproductive years, it is particularly important to rule out pregnancy. However, the absence of any urinary symptoms and the fact that she is not sexually active tend to make these pathologies less likely. The two most likely etiologies in this case are **gastroenteritis** or **appendicitis.** Unfortunately, it is often incredibly difficult to differentiate between these two etiologies initially. In this case, time may be a critical diagnostic tool. Observation is an important diagnostic tool in the evaluation of abdominal pain. This patient should be instructed to monitor her symptoms closely and contact her physician if her condition changes.

CASE 2-4

INITIAL PRESENTATION

The 38-year-old woman in Case 2-3 returns to the emergency department 8 hours later complaining of worsening pain and vomiting. She vomited once roughly 2 hours after her initial visit. Her pain is now localized to the right lower quadrant and is worsened by movement. She now notes chills.

PHYSICAL EXAMINATION

Her temperature is now 102.6°F, and her abdomen is extremely tender to even slight palpation, particularly in the right lower quadrant. There is involuntary guarding and prominent rebound tenderness.

LABORATORY TESTS

Laboratory testing includes a CBC significant for leukocytosis. Her electrolyte levels are normal.

ASSESSMENT

The patient now has localized pain, involuntary guarding, pain exacerbation with movement, and rebound tenderness. All of these signs and symptoms suggest parietal peritoneal involvement. The fever and leukocytosis are further evidence of significant inflammation. If this woman were sexually active, an ectopic pregnancy would be a strong possibility. A pregnancy test should be performed despite the negative history. This is a typical presentation for **appendicitis.** However, at this point, the actual diagnosis is considerably less relevant than the management plan. As a general rule, a surgical consult is necessary whenever there is evidence of peritoneal involvement, regardless of the presumptive diagnosis. Roughly one-fifth of surgical explorations for suspected appendicitis are negative, but this rate is considered acceptable because further delay may result in perforation and sepsis if appendicitis exists. A surgical consult is therefore warranted to rule out the diagnosis. If the surgeon proceeds with a laparotomy, one of several conditions may be found. Acute appendicitis is most likely, but Meckel's diverticulitis, although less common, is impossible to distinguish from appendicitis on clinical grounds. Acute pelvic inflammatory disease, ruptured endometrioma, a ruptured graafian follicle, or a twisted ovarian cyst are other possibilities in a woman this age.

The clinical diagnosis of appendicitis is even less certain in children who may have mesenteric adenitis or acute infectious gastroenteritis that may present with similar findings. The diagnosis is also more difficult in the elderly. They are prone to acute mesenteric thrombosis, diverticulitis, intestinal obstruction, and cholecystitis, all of which may mimic acute appendicitis.

Many of these conditions may be cured by the appropriate surgical procedure during the laparotomy, even if the problem was not the prime consideration prior to surgery. Other diagnoses may be made at laparotomy, which require different therapeutic modalities, such as antibiotics. A small percentage of patients have a negative laparotomy, no diagnosis made, and fully recover.

This woman had sufficient evidence to warrant a laparotomy. At surgery, an inflamed appendix was resected, and she recovered uneventfully.

CASE 2-5

INITIAL PRESENTATION

A 36-year-old woman who has had rheumatoid arthritis for 12 years is complaining of new onset abdominal pain that has persisted for 3 months. She describes a "burning" pain in the epigastric region that is aggravated by food. She has lost 6 lbs in the past 3 months. Her medications include indomethacin and corticosteroids. She occasionally has dark-colored stools.

PHYSICAL EXAMINATION

An abdominal examination reveals a soft abdomen with mild epigastric tenderness but no masses or bruits. A rectal examination is positive for occult blood.

ASSESSMENT

As with the other cases, localization may be somewhat helpful. Pain in the epigastric region can result from a disorder of the stomach, gallbladder, pancreas, small intestine, abdominal aorta, and occasionally, the esophagus or pleura. The presence of occult blood and history of melena help confirm involvement of the upper GI tract. In addition, the timing of this disorder is important. Obviously, this is a chronic condition, making infection, obstruction, or vessel disease less likely. Medication history is always an important part of the clinical picture but, in this case, it is particularly significant. Both nonsteroidal anti-inflammatory drugs (NSAIDs), such as indomethacin, and corticosteroids put this patient at a higher risk for PUD and gastritis.

This patient probably has **PUD** or **gastritis with bleeding,** and her medications may be contributing. She should undergo upper endoscopy. If this procedure confirms the suspected diagnosis, a regimen for healing the condition and preventing the recurrence should be instituted. Histamine-2 blockers are effective in healing, but misoprostol may be necessary to prevent recurrences if the rheumatoid arthritis mandates continued use of NSAIDs or corticosteroids.

If the upper endoscopy does not confirm a specific diagnosis, there is still a reasonable probability that the abdominal pain and bleeding are a result of medications, and the same treatment plan should be adopted. Further diagnostic studies at this point are unnecessary.

CASE 2-6

INITIAL PRESENTATION

A 73-year-old man complains of "indigestion" and "heartburn" since awakening this morning. The pain has been persistent for 3 hours, and there are no other associated symptoms. He had a

regular dinner the previous night, and this pain is new for the patient. His history includes hypertension for 40 years and a 55-pack-year history of smoking. The only medication he takes is lisinopril to control his blood pressure.

PHYSICAL EXAMINATION

The patient's blood pressure is 144/92 mm Hg, and his pulse is 88 beats/min and regular. He appears distressed. The remainder of the physical examination is within normal limits. An electrocardiogram (ECG) indicates ST-segment depression in leads I, II, aVL, V_3, V_4, V_5, and V_6.

ASSESSMENT

ST-segment depression on an ECG tracing is an indication of subendocardial ischemia. The patient's history of hypertension and smoking are risk factors for **coronary artery disease.** This case is included here to illustrate the importance of considering cardiac causes for patients presenting with apparent GI symptoms, particularly when significant risk factors are present. Like historical or laboratory data, risk factor data affect the probability that an individual has a certain diagnosis. When coupled with objective findings, such as ECG abnormalities, the case becomes even stronger. A first episode of heartburn at age 73 years would be very rare, whereas angina may certainly begin at that age. Unfortunately, coronary symptoms masquerading as GI problems are not uncommon, and missing the diagnosis can be catastrophic. In this case, angina was considered, and an ECG was performed. The abnormal ECG demands further investigation, and a coronary angiogram is probably indicated.

CASE 2-7

INITIAL PRESENTATION

An 86-year-old man presents with the complaint of left-sided abdominal pain for the past 5 days. He describes the pain as severe and burning, with the skin over the area of pain hypersensitive to touch. A rash appeared this morning in the region of the pain. There are no other associated symptoms.

PHYSICAL EXAMINATION

Physical examination reveals a left-sided rash extending from the middle of the back to the umbilicus in the area of the T9 or

T10 dermatome. The rash consists of small vesicles with an erythematous base.

ASSESSMENT

In this case, the acute onset, quality of pain, location, and associated rash are all very helpful diagnostic cues. Burning pain with hyperesthesia is always a hint that peripheral nerves may be involved. There are also no other associated symptoms that would indicate any other organ involvement. In addition, the dermatomal distribution in association with the rash indicates that this patient is most likely suffering from **herpes zoster virus (HZV).** The herpes virus lies dormant in sensory nerve ganglia after an initial infection with HZV (chicken pox). Herpes zoster is thought to be due to the reactivation of the virus due to advancing age, immunosuppression, or occasionally skin trauma. As the virus multiplies, the infection spreads along the nerves creating the characteristic dermatome of pain and usually clustered vesicles. It is important to note that pain often precedes and sometimes occurs without the presence of a rash. Unfortunately, antiviral therapy is only effective if given in the first day or two of the infection and, therefore, would not benefit this man. He can be given medication for pain control, and he should be observed for superinfection.

CASE 2-8

INITIAL PRESENTATION

A 34-year-old woman with type I diabetes mellitus (type I DM) complains of dull, left-sided abdominal pain that began 24 hours ago and is progressively increasing. She has associated chills and a loss of appetite. The pain is described as "dull and achy" and radiates around to the middle of her lower back. She has a history of recurrent urinary tract infections.

PHYSICAL EXAMINATION

The patient's temperature is 102.6°F, and she appears acutely ill. Left costovertebral angle tenderness is noted. The abdomen is soft with no masses or bruits. Bowel sounds are normal, but there is diffuse tenderness to palpation on the left side.

LABORATORY TESTS

Laboratory results include a WBC count of 14,000 (normal: 5000–10,000 µL), and urinalysis is positive for protein and leuko-

cyte esterase. Microscopic examination reveals many WBCs, red blood cells, and WBC casts.

ASSESSMENT

The acute onset and fever are consistent with an infectious etiology, and type I DM is a predisposing factor. Localization to the left side and radiation to the back suggests kidney involvement, a hypothesis that is more likely with the history of recurrent urinary tract infections. The urinalysis strongly supports an infectious process. As discussed earlier, the parenchyma of abdominal and retroperitoneal organs are not well innervated by sensory neurons. Inflammatory processes are sensed by organ capsules, resulting in dull, achy pain that is not usually localized or sharp until the well-innervated peritoneum becomes involved. This case is another example of abdominal pain resulting from a non-GI pathology. The most likely diagnosis for this patient is **pyelonephritis.** Further studies include blood and urine cultures, testing for sensitivity to antibiotics, and levels of blood urea nitrogen and creatinine. The patient will receive trimethoprim/sulfamethoxazole intravenously until sensitivity studies or lack of clinical improvement dictate a change. Meperidine may be necessary to control pain. Fluid status will be carefully monitored to ensure adequate urine output.

SUMMARY

Abdominal pain can result from a variety of very different pathologic processes. In addition, it is often difficult to make a definitive diagnosis of a patient with abdominal pain without invasive procedures such as surgery. However, the history and physical examination can be helpful in determining the probable diagnoses and in selecting the appropriate diagnostic procedures. The approach to the patient with abdominal pain must include an analysis of timing, associated symptoms, quality, quantity, location, and risk factors. Localization and quality of the pain can help indicate the type of pathology and the organ system involved. Unfortunately, referred pain occasionally confounds this approach, as discussed in Case 2-7. A classic example is pain referred to the shoulder from gallbladder or splenic disorders. The following are very general guidelines for types of abdominal pain and the possible problem:

- "Colicky" or cramping pain indicates smooth muscle spasm or obstruction.
- Sharp, well-defined pain exacerbated by movement usually indicates involvement of the parietal peritoneum.
- Burning pain is often a sign of mucosal irritation, as in PUD.
- Severe burning pain with hyperesthesia is often indicative of a peripheral sensory nerve disturbance.

- Dull pain may be a sign of increased pressure on an organ capsule.

Analysis of timing may be very helpful in the diagnostic process. Acute pain is usually infectious, vascular, or obstructive in origin. Chronic pain indicates pathologies with slower, more indolent progressions such as some systemic disorders, chronic inflammation, or neoplastic processes. Associated factors such as fever, jaundice, appetite or diet changes, blood in stools, aggravation by food, or changes in the pattern of urination can also aid the differential diagnosis. Physical examination of the abdomen can be helpful if masses are present or if the patient has peritoneal involvement. The physical examination also can be helpful to document associated factors such as jaundice or occult blood in stools. Unfortunately, as in the case of appendicitis, definitive diagnosis may not be possible without surgery. However, the history and the physical examination can at least help to determine when surgical or other invasive procedures are indicated.

CHAPTER 3
Chief Complaint: Shortness of Breath

- -

CASE 3-1

INITIAL PRESENTATION

Mrs. M., a 56-year-old office manager, presents to a clinic with a chief complaint of shortness of breath during the past 3 years. Upon questioning, the following information is revealed. Mrs. M. first noticed shortness of breath when doing light housework roughly 3 years ago. Since that time, she feels that it has been getting "really bad" and reports difficulty walking up a flight of stairs without "gasping for air." During the past few weeks, she has been having some difficulty breathing even at rest. She also reports a persistent dry cough, which has worsened during the past 4 years. Mrs. M. states that she has not been coughing up mucus or blood. She denies wheezing, chest pain, lightheadedness when standing or walking, edema, and fever. She says that she has never awakened at night with difficulty breathing. She has smoked two packs of cigarettes a day for the past 20 years. She does not drink alcohol or use drugs. She is not aware of any exposure to harmful toxins or chemicals. She has no other medical problems of which she is aware. She has no history of dark stools or rectal bleeding. She is postmenopausal and denies any vaginal bleeding. She does not exercise on a regular basis. She has no history of trauma or injury. She states that she has not been overly anxious and describes her mood as generally "good."

> Progressively worsening chronic dyspnea

> Associated dry cough

> No evidence of cardiac involvement or fever

> No paroxysmal nocturnal dyspnea

> Risk factors

> No signs of blood loss or anemia.

1. What organ systems can be involved in the pathogenesis of dyspnea (in any patient)?
2. How has the patient's history helped to develop a list of reasonable hypotheses?

Discussion

Dyspnea refers to the unpleasant sensation of difficult breathing and suggests one of the following: (1) stimulation of chemoreceptors by decreased oxygen levels or a build-up of carbon dioxide; (2) stimulation of mechanoreceptors in the airways and chest wall; or (3) activation of outgoing respiratory motor command signals from the central nervous system (CNS). When approaching a patient with dyspnea, the systems summarized in Table 3-1 could be involved.

TABLE 3-1
SYSTEMS POTENTIALLY INVOLVED IN PATIENTS WITH DYSPNEA

System	Possible Causes
Pulmonary	Pneumonia
	Chronic obstructive pulmonary disease
	Idiopathic pulmonary fibrosis, via stimulation of chemoreceptors and mechanoreceptors
Cardiac	Congestive heart failure
	Myocardial infarction via stimulation of chemoreceptors (However, if "backward" failure is prominent enough, pulmonary edema may result and stimulate pulmonary mechanoreceptors.)
Hematologic	Anemia via chemoreceptor stimulation as a result of inadequate hemoglobin to transport sufficient oxygen
Metabolic	Acidosis[a]
Psychological	Anxiety (disorders such as acute anxiety attacks may cause dyspnea via altered CNS-controlled respiratory regulation.)
CNS	Trauma or cerebrovascular accident, which may alter CNS-controlled respiratory regulation
Musculoskeletal	Fractured rib or strained muscle in chest wall via direct stimulation of mechanoreceptors and by inhibiting patient's ability to take a deep breath
Peripheral nervous system	Myasthenia gravis, Lambert-Eaton syndrome, and other disorders that compromise the ability to expand the chest

[a] Excess hydrogen in metabolic acidosis increases carbon dioxide via the carbonic anhydrase-catalyzed reaction: $H^+ + HCO_3^- \leftrightarrow H_2CO_3 \leftrightarrow H_2O + CO_2$. Increased levels of carbon dioxide and hydrogen then stimulate chemoreceptors, resulting in rapid, deep breathing. This breathing pattern decreases carbon dioxide, shifts the equation to the right, and thus decreases hydrogen.

Exertional dyspnea suggests a lack of oxygen delivery or a carbon dioxide build-up. The presence of a cough suggests pulmonary involvement, either directly or indirectly. This patient's cough is nonproductive. This fact, the chronic nature of her illness, and the absence of fever all tend to rule out an infectious etiology. However, other pulmonary pathologies such as emphysema, asthma, and idiopathic pulmonary fibrosis (IPF) are still possibilities. In addition, the patient's cough reflex could be stimulated because of pulmonary congestion secondary to left-sided heart failure. Obviously, forward failure would also result in decreased oxygen delivery, increased carbon dioxide build-up, and thus dyspnea. However, the absence of chest pain, orthopnea, paroxysmal nocturnal dyspnea (PND), and edema all suggest a lack of cardiac involvement. This patient's smoking could contribute to both cardiac and pulmonary causes of her illness. There is nothing in her history, such as excessive bleeding or overexercise (e.g., jogger's anemia), that might indicate anemia as a cause of her problems. She has no known exposure to respiratory toxins, which helps rule out problems such as asbestosis. This patient has no other medical problems, which, along with the chronic and progressive nature of her symptoms, makes a metabolic disorder (e.g., diabetic ketoacidosis) less likely. The absence of trauma either to the chest or to the head points away from either a musculoskeletal or a CNS disorder. There is no evidence at this point of an anxiety disorder. All of this information points to a pulmonary etiology, although a cardiac cause cannot yet be dismissed.

PHYSICAL EXAMINATION

Mrs. M.'s vital signs are: blood pressure, 116/70 mm Hg (supine) and 114/72 mm Hg (standing); pulse, 76 beats/min (supine) and 84 beats/min (standing); and respiration rate, 20 breaths/min. Her lungs are slightly hyperresonant to percussion. There is no wheezing, but there are inspiratory crackles at both bases. A cardiac examination reveals a normal first heart sound (S_1), a physiologically split second heart sound (S_2), and no gallops. There is no cyanosis in the extremities; digital clubbing is noted bilaterally. The remainder of the physical examination is unremarkable.

3. How does this information help modify the list of possible diagnoses?
4. What laboratory tests should be ordered for this patient?

Discussion

It is significant that the pulse rate and blood pressure are within normal limits. This helps to confirm that Mrs. M. does not have longstanding hypertension leading to congestive heart failure (CHF) and indicates that her problem is not yet severe enough to cause her heart rate to increase dramatically. More important, however, is the fact that she has no evidence of orthostatic hypotension (i.e., when moving from a supine to a standing position, an increase in heart rate of 20–30 beats/min, a fall in systolic blood pressure greater than 20–30 mm Hg, or a fall in diastolic blood pressure greater than 10–15 mm Hg). In this case the heart is responding appropriately to changes in position. The respiratory rate of 20 breaths/min is at the upper limits of normal and supports the idea that this woman is having difficulty acquiring oxygen or blowing off carbon dioxide. The abnormal lung examination further supports a pulmonary etiology for this woman's problem, and the normal cardiac examination and absence of cyanosis and edema both help to rule out a cardiac etiology. Although the exact mechanism is unknown, digital clubbing is most likely the result of hormonal changes secondary to pulmonary problems. Overall, the physical examination helps to confirm a pulmonary problem in this patient. Therefore, it is reasonable to order laboratory tests that help differentiate among pulmonary problems. It is important to be as efficient as possible, without compromising the patient's safety or comfort.

A chest radiograph, arterial blood gases (ABGs), and pulmonary function tests (PFTs) are ordered. Perhaps more information units per dollar spent are provided by a chest radiograph than by any other diagnostic test. A chest radiograph can rule out many congenital and structural problems of the heart and lungs as well as infections, neoplasms, and traumatic effects. It gives us a superb anatomic view of the chest with no risk or discomfort to the patient. ABGs provide information as to the effectiveness of respiration by measuring those substances that are brought into the body and those that are expelled by the lungs and, to some degree, by the kidneys. PFTs demonstrate the mechanical ability of the lungs to move air. These three tests—chest radiograph, ABGs, and PFTs—usually can determine whether dyspnea is psychologic, pulmonary, cardiac, or metabolic in origin.

LABORATORY TESTS

The chest radiograph shows diffuse, bilateral, ground-glass infiltrates. The laboratory test results are provided in the table below.

Laboratory Tests	Patient	Normal Values
Arterial blood gases		
pH	7.43	7.38–7.44
Partial pressure of carbon dioxide (P_{CO_2})	29 mm Hg	35–45 mm Hg
Partial pressure of oxygen (P_{O_2})	81 mm Hg	80–100 mm Hg
Bicarbonate (HCO_3^-)	22 mEq/L	21–30 mEq/L

Laboratory Tests	Patient	Predicted Values
Pulmonary function tests		
Forced vital capacity (FVC)	2.30 L	3.26 L
Forced expiratory volume in 1 second (FEV_1)	2.02 L	2.59 L
FEV_1/FVC	88%	79%

5. How should the results of the ABGs be interpreted?
6. How should the results of the PFTs be interpreted?
7. How do the test results help form a diagnosis?

Discussion

The ABGs indicate a compensated respiratory alkalosis. The low P_{CO_2} and low-normal P_{O_2} suggest hyperpnea. As a response to decreased blood oxygenation, the patient is breathing faster or deeper. The hyperpnea lowers P_{CO_2}, and this causes respiratory alkalosis. The kidneys have had time to correct the alkalosis, and thus the pH is normal.

The PFTs indicate a restrictive pattern without evidence of obstruction. This obviously eliminates chronic obstructive pulmonary disease (COPD) as a cause. Therefore, this woman has a restrictive lung disease characterized by difficulty with oxygenation and diffuse ground-glass infiltrates on chest radiograph. Although a biopsy is necessary to establish a definitive diagnosis, these findings are consistent with pulmonary fibrosis. Because there is no known history of exposure to respiratory toxins for this patient, the most likely diagnosis is idiopathic pulmonary fibrosis.

ASSESSMENT

This woman appears to have **idiopathic pulmonary fibrosis**. Her management plan includes an open lung biopsy to prove the diagnosis. Without this procedure, diseases such as eosinophilic granuloma, hypersensitivity pneumonitis, and lymphangiomyomatosis may be mistakenly diagnosed as IPF. Treatment is different for these disorders, so a firm diagnosis is imperative. The management of IPF is mostly supportive, with the use of bronchodilators if there is any element of bronchospasm and supplemental oxygen if the hypoxemia is severe. Pneumococcal and influenza immunizations are essential in patients such as Mrs. M. who have compromised lung function.

CASE 3-2

INITIAL PRESENTATION

A 32-year-old man presents complaining of shortness of breath. He reports experiencing dyspnea with minimal exercise for the past 2 months that has been gradually getting worse. He has had orthopnea for the past 2 weeks. He states that he has a nonproductive cough when recumbent. Pitting edema has been present for 2 weeks. He has no fever or chest pain. His medical history is negative except for heavy alcohol intake that was greater than 1 pint of whiskey a day for 5 years, until quitting 3 weeks ago.

PHYSICAL EXAMINATION

The patient appears thin and chronically ill. He shows no cyanosis. A cardiac examination reveals an third heart sound (S_3) gallop.

LABORATORY TESTS

There is 2+ pitting ankle edema and no ascites. A chest radiograph indicates diffuse cardiac enlargement, and his electrocardiogram (ECG) is low voltage. Laboratory test results are as follows:

Laboratory Tests	Patient	Normal Values
Bilirubin (total)	0.6 mg/dL	0.3–1.1 mg/dL
Albumin	3.9 g/dL	3.3–5.2 g/dL
Aspartate aminotransferase (AST)	74 U/L	1–36 U/L
Prothrombin time (PT)	23 sec	12.0–14.0 sec
Hematocrit	32%	35%–45%
Mean cell volume	105 fL	80–100 fL

8. What is meant by a low-voltage ECG, and what are the likely causes?

Discussion

A low-voltage ECG means that the waves on the ECG tracing are not very high or low. This is caused by insulation (e.g., fluid, fat, air) between the heart and the ECG lead. Like Mrs. M. (see Case 3-1), this patient is complaining of dyspnea and is experiencing progressively worsening, exertional dyspnea. Thus, pulmonary, hematologic, or cardiac etiologies are suspected. Unlike Mrs. M., however, this individual has orthopnea, a cough when recumbent, and edema. These conditions suggest that fluid has accumulated in the lungs and lower extremities, which occurs when the heart is unable to pump blood out of the venous systems into the arterial systems. Thus, dyspnea in this case is more likely caused by CHF. The S_3 noted on physical examination further supports this diagnosis. In addition, congestion in both the lower extremities (right side) and pulmonary vasculature (left side) indicate that this patient is suffering from biventricular heart failure. This is helpful in the diagnosis because heart failure secondary to longstanding hypertension would present initially as left-sided failure only. Another important feature of this patient's presentation is his relatively young age. CHF is most common in elderly people with ischemic myocardial disease. Because this man is not elderly, there must be another cause for his condition. The only other significant problem he has is a history of alcoholism.

9. Could this patient's alcoholism and CHF be related?

The presence of the signs and symptoms of CHF usually means the patient has CHF, even in the absence of strongly associated risk factors (e.g., age). While it is possible for a patient to have several unrelated problems, it is reasonable to look for relationships between two apparently separate conditions. A significant risk history, such as alcohol abuse in this case, makes one suspicious of possible health problems. In fact, there is a relationship between excessive alcohol use and CHF.

ASSESSMENT

This patient is most likely suffering from **alcoholic cardiomyopathy**. He has CHF secondary to alcoholism. This patient will be given a diuretic for initial treatment, and he will be referred to a cardiologist. The physician will educate the patient about the causes of CHF and will reinforce the patient's need for continued abstinence from alcohol.

CASE 3-3

INITIAL PRESENTATION

A 23-year-old woman complains of decreasing exercise tolerance due to shortness of breath and fatigue during the past 2 months. She reports no cough, fever, or exposure to fumes or excessive respiratory pollutants, and no paroxysmal nocturnal PND or orthopnea. She has no history of tobacco, alcohol, or drug use. She jogs regularly but cannot run as fast as she had previously. Her medical and family histories are unremarkable.

PHYSICAL EXAMINATION

The physician notes a healthy-appearing young woman with no obvious respiratory abnormalities. All her vital signs are normal, but a cardiac examination reveals a II/VI systolic murmur. The remainder of the examination is normal.

ASSESSMENT

This patient has exertional dyspnea, as did the patients in Cases 3-1 and 3-2, and, like the man with alcoholic cardiomyopathy, this patient has a noted abnormal heart sound. Like the others, this patient has no fever that might indicate an infectious process. However, this patient has no cough or other indications of pulmonary involvement. She also has no indication of significant cardiac failure, such as PND or orthopnea. There is nothing in her risk factor assessment that presents concern, as it did for the patient with alcoholism or for Mrs. M., who smoked. In summary, this patient is not a typical presentation of a cardiac or pulmonary etiology as were the patients in Cases 3-1 and 3-2. As stated in Case 3-2, dyspnea may be caused by stimulation of chemoreceptors due to a decrease in oxygen level or a build-up of carbon dioxide. Thus, any break in the chain of oxygen delivery and carbon dioxide removal, such as a defect in the transportation of these gases, could be a cause of dyspnea. There is a fine but potentially important distinction between this patient's presentation and those of the other two: This patient is not complaining of exertional dyspnea but rather decreased exercise tolerance and fatigue. These symptoms suggest anemia as the primary cause of her complaints, and the II/VI systolic murmur is consistent with this hypothesis. Anemia results in decreased oxygen delivery to peripheral tissues. The body responds by increasing the heart rate to increase cardiac output. The increased heart rate often results in turbulent blood flow and a so-called flow murmur. Knowing a patient's age and habits are helpful when trying to differentiate diagnoses. First, this woman is young, so pulmonary or cardiac problems are unlikely in the absence of other risk factors. She is also premenopausal and exercises regularly; thus, iron deficiency anemia from menstrual blood loss and increased iron needs from exercise is not unlikely.

This woman is given a presumptive diagnosis of **iron deficiency anemia** indicated by dyspnea with exercise and a systolic heart murmur. Measurement of hematocrit, hemoglobin, mean corpuscular volume (MCV), serum iron, and TIBC levels will be ordered. If these tests confirm a classic microcytic, hypochromic anemia of iron deficiency, she will be placed on 300 mg of oral iron a day. Once her hematocrit level has returned to normal and her bone marrow iron stores have been replenished, a low maintenance dose of iron supplementation will be considered.

CASE 3-4

INITIAL PRESENTATION

A 72-year-old woman with diabetes mellitus complains of shortness of breath. Her symptoms began abruptly 1 day ago with shaking chills and high fever following a "cold" that lasted for 1 week. She has an associated cough with rust-colored sputum and associated right-sided pleuritic chest pain. There is no edema, orthopnea, or PND. The woman has a 30-pack-year history of smoking.

PHYSICAL EXAMINATION

The patient's temperature is 103°F, her pulse is 110 beats/min, her respirations are 28 breaths/min, and her blood pressure is 140/70 mm Hg. A lung examination is significant for rales, decreased breath sounds, dullness to percussion, increased fremitus (increased vibrations carried from the larynx to the chest wall), and "ee-to-ay changes" noted in the right lower lobe.

ASSESSMENT

As in Cases 3-1 and 3-2, this patient has some high-risk factors. She is elderly, diabetic, and has a smoking history, all of which place this patient at high risk for cardiac and pulmonary disease. However, this case has several strikingly different aspects. First, this patient's symptoms began acutely. Also, she notes a high fever. These two factors suggest an infectious process. As in Cases 3-1 and

3-3, the absence of edema, PND, and orthopnea help to rule out a cardiac etiology. In addition, this patient's pleuritic chest pain and cough productive of rust-colored sputum suggest a pulmonary etiology. Her elevated temperature is consistent with her history of a recent infection. The lung examination reinforces a right lower lobe pathology. Furthermore, specific examination findings of increased fremitus, decreased breath sounds, and dullness to percussion suggest pulmonary consolidation.

This is a good example of a physical examination that differentiates between two etiologies. Dullness to percussion and decreased breath sounds indicate a somewhat solid area that is not being used for respiration. However, these findings do not distinguish between a pulmonary parenchymal etiology (e.g., pneumonia) and a pleural pathology (e.g., effusion). Rales, on the other hand, are produced by the opening and closing of alveoli; thus, it is reasonable to assume that the pulmonary parenchyma is involved. In addition, fremitus is increased when pulmonary consolidation is present because the consolidation provides a medium through which sound waves can travel. However, a pleural effusion acts as a barrier to the transmission of sound waves because the vibrating parenchyma is pushed further away from the chest wall and thus the stethoscope. Altogether, this patient's history and physical examination strongly suggest a diagnosis of **pneumonia**, the most likely type being pneumococcal. She will undergo a chest radiograph and sputum and blood cultures. The patient will begin a course of a broad-spectrum antibiotic pending results of the cultures.

SUMMARY

Reduced to the basics, dyspnea is a warning that the body has a problem that might be ameliorated with deeper or faster breathing. Table 3-1 lists the multiple systems that may trigger the symptom of dyspnea. Although there are many causes of this disturbing feeling, a careful analysis of the patient's symptoms, signs, and risk factors can quickly narrow the diagnostic focus.

CHAPTER 4
Chief Complaint: High Cholesterol

CASE 4-1

INITIAL PRESENTATION

Mr. D. is a 26-year-old man who presents because he recently had his cholesterol checked at the mall and was told that it was 230 mg/dL. Mr. D. does not smoke, drink, or use drugs. He has no history of diabetes, kidney disease, liver disease, or hypothyroidism. He also takes no medications on a regular basis. He states that he has never had high blood pressure, heart problems, or episodes of pancreatitis. Mr. D. reports that his father recently died of a heart attack in his late forties, but says his family is otherwise "pretty healthy." He states that he exercises regularly but does not like to eat "all that health food stuff"; his diet consists mainly of fast food and frozen dinners. He rarely eats fruits or vegetables and never eats fish.

> Primary hyper-cholesterolemia

> No manifestations

> Possible familial disorder

1. How should this patient be managed?
2. Which lipid levels are risk factors for Mr. D.?

Discussion

Mr. D. comes to the clinic with an elevated cholesterol level based on a test from the mall. The first question to ask is how accurate is the cholesterol test from the mall. The answer is somewhat. The major concern here is that a possible lipid disorder could lead to coronary artery disease (CAD). However, the ability of total cholesterol screening to identify high-risk individuals has been found to be low in the general population. Therefore, it is extremely important to consider the pretest probability of this patient having a lipid disorder.

Mr. D. is an apparently healthy individual. There is nothing in his personal history, such as chronic illnesses or medication use, that could contribute to an increased cholesterol level. Of concern, however, is the fact that his father died at a relatively young age of a heart attack. This indicates that the patient may suffer from a familial lipid disorder and that he could be at risk for CAD due to other inherited factors. In this case, it is important to rule out any compounding problems, such as an elevated cholesterol level.

PHYSICAL EXAMINATION

> No physical evidence of a lipid disorder

Examination reveals a thin, healthy-appearing man in no apparent distress. He is normotensive. He has no xanthomas. His cardiac examination is normal, and no carotid bruits are noted.

LABORATORY TESTS

Mr. D.'s laboratory results are listed below.

Laboratory Tests	Patient	Normal Values
Total cholesterol	240 mg/dL	< 200 mg/dL (ideally)
Triglycerides	195 mg/dL	40–200 mg/dL
High-density lipoprotein (HDL)	34 mg/dL	> 35 mg/dL (ideally)
Low-density lipoprotein (LDL)[a]	167 mg/dL	62–165 mg/dL

[a] LDL = total cholesterol − HDL − (triglycerides/5).

3. Assuming secondary causes of hyperlipidemia are ruled out, what should be done now?
4. What medication should this patient be prescribed if pharmacologic intervention becomes necessary?

Discussion

This patient has laboratory evidence of increased total cholesterol, an LDL level at the upper end of normal, a slightly low HDL level, and a relatively normal level of triglycerides. Given his father's cardiac history and the patient's lack of other contributing factors, he is most likely suffering from familial hypercholesterolemia. The most important goal of treatment is to decrease his cholesterol to prevent the long-term effects of the disorder, such as CAD. The first step in management of a primary hyperlipidemia should always include diet and risk factor control. In particular, this patient should be encouraged to increase his intake of fruits and vegetables and decrease his intake of fats. Although the consumption of fish may actually increase LDL levels, it may help prevent the long-term effects of elevated LDL, such as CAD. If dietary manipulation proves ineffective, pharmacologic intervention may be necessary.

There are many choices for pharmacologic intervention in the treatment of lipid disorders. This patient does not have elevated triglycerides, but he does have a relatively high level of LDL. In addition, his HDL level is slightly low. HDL is important for removing cholesterol from peripheral tissues, and low levels of HDL may increase the risk of CAD. Niacin would be appropriate because it is effective for lowering LDL and raising HDL. In addition, niacin is the only agent shown to decrease levels of lipoprotein(a) effectively, which is believed to play a role in the pathogenesis of CAD. The most common side effect of niacin is flushing, which can usually be alleviated with aspirin. Other side effects include gastrointestinal upset, hepatitis, and hyperuricemia. Bile acid resins, such as cholestyramine, would be another appropriate choice for this patient because they are effective in lowering LDL. Unfortunately, these drugs do not increase HDL levels, and the major side effects of constipation and indigestion can reduce patient compliance. Similarly, hydroxymethylglutaryl–coenzyme A (HMG-CoA) reductase inhibitors, such as lovastatin, lower LDL but do not significantly increase the HDL levels. However, the ratio of HDL to LDL is most important, so any reduction of LDL and increase in HDL should reduce the risk of CAD.

ASSESSMENT

This patient has **hypercholesterolemia** with an adverse HDL/LDL ratio, which places him at risk for developing coronary and other arterial diseases if left untreated. If diet changes prove ineffective, niacin, 1 g orally three times a day, should be prescribed. Lipids should be checked in 4-6 weeks, and the dose of niacin adjusted accordingly.

CASE 4-2

INITIAL PRESENTATION

A 56-year-old man with type II diabetes mellitus (type II DM) is referred for evaluation of his lipid disorder. His medications include 20 mg of glyburide per day. His glucose level averages 360 mg/dL per home glucose meter. He has no history of heart problems or pancreatitis. He describes his diet as "poor."

PHYSICAL EXAMINATION

The patient's height is 6′0″, his weight is 260 lbs, his pulse is 70 beats/min, his blood pressure is 140/80 mm Hg, and he is afebrile.

LABORATORY TESTS

Laboratory results are listed in the table below.

Laboratory Tests	Patient	Normal Values
Total cholesterol	216 mg/dL	< 200 mg/dL
Triglycerides	420 mg/dL	40–200 mg/dL
HDL	30 mg/dL	> 35 mg/dL
LDL (calculated)	102 mg/dL	< 130 mg/dL
HbA_{1c}	11.6%	5.6%–7.5%

HbA_{1c} = glycosylated hemoglobin.

ASSESSMENT

As with Mr. D. in Case 4-1, this patient has some lipid abnormalities. However, unlike Mr. D., this person most likely has a **secondary lipid disorder due to his diabetes**. Patients with diabetes frequently have increased levels of triglycerides combined with increased levels of total cholesterol or decreased levels of HDL. In this case, the patient's hemoglobin A_{1c} (HbA_{1c}) and reported glucose meter readings indicate that his diabetes is not in good control. Management of this patient's lipid disorder first requires control of his diabetes. Unfortunately, he is already on a high dose of glyburide. Possible options include adding a biguanide such as metformin or considering one of the new peripheral insulin-sensitizing agents, such as troglitazone. Also, this patient is clearly overweight, so a diet and exercise program should be considered. Patients often describe their diet as "poor." It is difficult to know what this means without further inquiry, but it is clear that this patient should be on a low-fat, diabetic diet. Weight loss should help increase this patient's insulin sensitivity and eventually help to decrease his lipid levels. If glucose control, diet manipulation, and exercise strategies prove unsuccessful in correcting this patient's lipid disorder, one of the fibrates (e.g., gemfibrozil) would be an effective agent for lowering his triglyceride level, and it could be combined with a bile acid resin to decrease LDL, if necessary. Niacin should be avoided in patients with diabetes because of its potential for exacerbating hyperglycemia.

CASE 4-3

INITIAL PRESENTATION

A 44-year-old woman complains of increased fatigue and cold intolerance during the past 2 months. She has no history of heart problems or pancreatitis. The patient reports a 20-lb weight gain during the past 3–4 months.

PHYSICAL EXAMINATION

The woman's hair is brittle and dry, and her skin is notably dry. Her reflexes are 2+ with a slow return bilaterally in all extremities.

LABORATORY TESTS

The patient's laboratory results are listed below.

Laboratory Tests	Patient	Normal Values
Total cholesterol	304 mg/dL	< 200 mg/dL
Triglycerides	192 mg/dL	40–200 mg/dL
HDL	44 mg/dL	> 35 mg/dL
LDL (calculated)	222 mg/dL	62–165 mg/dL

ASSESSMENT

As with the other patients, this individual has elevated cholesterol. In this case, the major anomaly appears to be the LDL cholesterol. If isolated elevation of LDL were this patient's only problem, pharmacologic intervention would be relatively simple. Bile acid resins, HMG-CoA reductase inhibitors, probucol, and niacin would be reasonable choices. However, as with the patient in Case 4-2, this patient has evidence of a secondary disorder. The history of weight gain, fatigue, and cold intolerance, in addition to the physical examination findings of brittle hair, dry skin, and reflexes exhibiting a slow return, all suggest a diagnosis of **hypothyroidism**. Many patients with hypothyroidism also have increased levels of LDL, triglycerides, or both. Again, controlling the underlying disorder should be the first approach to treatment, once the diagnosis has been definitely determined with laboratory tests. Correcting the hypothyroidism should concomitantly correct the lipid abnormality.

CASE 4-4

INITIAL PRESENTATION

A 36-year-old man is referred for evaluation of recurrent pancreatitis. He has had three episodes of pancreatitis in the last 6 years, the last one 2 weeks ago. He has no history or symptoms of diabetes, thyroid disease, myeloma, kidney disease, biliary obstruction, or hepatitis. He has no history of alcohol use and is not currently on any medications. He has had difficulty maintaining a proper weight since childhood.

PHYSICAL EXAMINATION

The patient's height is 5′10″, and his weight is 195 lbs.; his temperature, pulse, and blood pressure are normal. There are multiple xanthomas present on his trunk and extremities.

LABORATORY TESTS

Laboratory values are given below.

Laboratory Tests	Patient	Normal Values
Total cholesterol	210 mg/dL	< 200 mg/dL
Triglycerides	560 mg/dL	40–200 mg/dL
HDL	33 mg/dL	> 35 mg/dL
LDL (calculated)	Unable to calculate when triglyceride level is higher than 500 mg/dL.	62–165 mg/dL
Glucose	83 mg/dL	70–115 mg/dL

ASSESSMENT

As in the case of Mr. D., this patient has no evidence of a secondary cause for his lipid disorder. Therefore, treatment should be directed toward correcting the specific lipid abnormality. Although diet and exercise should always be a part of any plan to correct a dyslipidemia, this patient probably has a significant genetic abnormality as a result of the dramatically increased triglycerides. The increased triglyceride level is the most likely cause for this patient's xanthomas and recurrent pancreatitis. The fibrates are the first-line pharmacologic therapy for hypertriglyceridemia. Niacin may be added if necessary. Unfortunately, the fibrates may increase LDL levels, and a bile acid resin may be needed to decrease levels of this lipoprotein. HMG-CoA reductase inhibitors should not be used in conjunction with the fibrates because of the increased risk of rhabdomyolysis and myopathy.

SUMMARY

Elevated lipid levels are frequently encountered in internal medicine. It is important to control lipids to help avoid long-term complications, such as CAD and pancreatitis. The approach to any patient with an apparent lipid disorder should always include a screening for other diseases that might adversely affect cholesterol, such as diabetes, hypothyroidism, kidney disease, or liver abnormalities. If any of these conditions are present, treatment should first be directed at the primary disorder. If a patient is found to have a primary lipid disorder, a diet and exercise plan, in addition to risk factor management, should be a part of the treatment plan. Finally, if pharmacologic intervention is required, it should be tailored to the individual's specific lipid disorder.

CHAPTER 5
Chief Complaint: Acute Chest Pain

CASE 5-1

INITIAL PRESENTATION

Mrs. M., a 72-year-old housewife, presents to the emergency department with chest pain. Mrs. M. states that approximately 4 hours ago, while taking her morning walk, she began having chest pain. The pain is described as a dull, substernal ache that radiates into her left arm and jaw. She tells the physician that the pain is moderately severe and seems to be getting worse. The pain is not affected by movement or deep inspiration, but it is relieved slightly when she rests. She has also noted slight shortness of breath and sweating during the last hour. Although she denies having any pain like this previously, Mrs. M. states that she has noticed slight chest discomfort when doing light housework during the past 2–3 months, but she dismissed it as "indigestion." Her medical history is significant for 20 years of high cholesterol, for which she is treated with the hydroxymethylglutaryl–coenzyme A (HMG-CoA) reductase inhibitor lovastatin, and 35 years of high blood pressure, for which she takes the calcium channel blocker diltiazem. Mrs. M. has a 65-pack-year history of smoking. She drinks no alcohol and takes no other drugs or medications. She is postmenopausal but does not take hormone replacement because her mother died of breast cancer at the age of 55. She has no family history of heart disease of which she is aware.

> Symptoms such as substernal chest pain radiating to the left arm and jaw are very suspicious for an acute cardiac event.

> Risk factors

Mrs. M. is happily married to Mr. M., who is a retired electrical engineer.

1. Does the radiation of the substernal pain to the left arm and jaw help to narrow the diagnostic possibilities?
2. What is the importance of the pain being unaffected by movement or deep inspiration?

Discussion

As with other complaints, chest pain may indicate a variety of diagnoses. The quality and nature of the pain, risk factors, and associated symptoms can be very helpful. Although many disorders may cause chest pain, the upper trunk of the body is relatively devoid of organs. Therefore, approaching a patient's problem from an organ system basis is often helpful and may quickly eliminate those etiologies that are immediately life-threatening. With some exceptions, pathology in the following structures can result in chest pain: the pericardium, myocardium, lungs, aorta, chest wall, and esophagus. Characteristics of the pain can rule out many etiologies initially. In this particular case, dull, aching pain not affected by movement or inspiration is indicative of organ parenchymal involvement, making pleural or pericardial involvement less likely. In addition, the patient's history of smoking, lack of hormone replacement, high cholesterol, high blood pressure, and the radiating nature of the pain make a primary cardiac problem highly likely. Esophageal problems often present similarly; however, esophageal disorders are usually not acutely life-threatening. Any presentation such as this requires the physician to rule out a cardiac problem before pursuing other pathologies.

PHYSICAL EXAMINATION

Mrs. M.'s vital signs are as follows: temperature, 100°F; blood pressure, 152/90 mm Hg; pulse, 88 beats/min, regular; height, 62″; and weight, 134 lbs. General appearance reveals a well-developed elderly woman who appears anxious and in some acute distress. Cardiac examination shows a regular rate without any murmurs, gallops, or rubs. The lungs are clear to percussion and auscultation. The remainder of the physical examination is within normal limits.

3. Would the essentially normal physical examination deter you from pursuing a cardiac etiology?

Discussion

Except for a third (S_3) and fourth (S_4) heart sound and diaphoresis, the physical examination may reveal little in a patient with an acute cardiac event. A chest radiograph may help reveal a chest abnormality, and it is usually indicated when chest pathology is suspected. The normal result provides little information in this case except that the patient does not have a pulmonary infiltrate, pleural effusion, or a collapsed lung.

LABORATORY TESTS

The patient's electrocardiogram (ECG) showed anterior ST-segment elevation, but her chest radiograph was normal. Other test results are given in the table below.

Laboratory Tests	Patient	Normal Values	Comments
Creatine kinase (CK)	122 U/L	90–140 U/L	Negative for acute myocardial damage
Lactate dehydrogenase (LDH)	155 U/L	95–200 U/L	Negative for acute myocardial damage
Aspartate aminotransferase (AST)	12 U/L	6–18 U/L	Negative for acute myocardial damage
Troponin I	0.65 ng/mL	0–0.69 ng/mL	Negative for acute myocardial infarction (MI)
		0.7–3.0 ng/mL	Possible cardiac damage 2–7 days prior
		> 3.0 ng/mL	Diagnostic of acute MI

4. How would you interpret these laboratory results?

Discussion

Enzyme levels can be extremely helpful in the diagnosis of cardiac ischemia. However, as with any test, sensitivity and specificity are an issue. CK is an enzyme found in skeletal muscle, cardiac muscle, and, to a much smaller extent, the brain. If this were elevated, the CK level would need to be fractionated into its isoenzymes to determine its origin. CK-MM is the most prominent isoenzyme; normal CK levels are virtually all CK-MM. This isoenzyme is found primarily in skeletal muscle. Cardiac muscle, on the other hand, is composed of both CK-MM and CK-MB. CK-BB is derived mainly from brain, gastrointestinal, and genitourinary tissue. Elevation of the CK-MB isoenzyme is indicative of cardiac injury. Similarly, LDH is found throughout the body, and fractionation is necessary to determine its origin. LDH_1 and LDH_2 are elevated after an MI. AST is found in a variety of tissues. Although it is not fractionated, elevation of AST in conjunction with clinical evidence can help rule in cardiac ischemia. The troponins are found in both skeletal and cardiac muscle. However, monoclonal antibodies to the troponin in cardiac muscle do not cross-react with the troponin in skeletal muscle. The troponin tests are relatively new; their effectiveness for ruling an MI in or out is presently being evaluated, but they appear to be more sensitive and specific than the other enzyme tests. In addition, elevated levels of troponin I may be better indicators of mortality following unstable angina or MI.

Unfortunately, none of these enzymes can be expected to be elevated in the first few hours following an MI (Table 5-1). Therefore, negative results do not rule out a cardiac event. The ECG tracing exhibiting anterior ST-segment elevation is consistent with an MI and should be followed up.

TABLE 5-1
ENZYMES ELEVATED AFTER MYOCARDIAL INFARCTION

Enzyme	First Increase	Time to Maximum	Relative Elevation
CK	3–6 hours	12–24 hours	6–8 times normal
LDH	12 hours	2–3 days	4–6 times normal
AST	8 hours	2–3 days	2–4 times normal
Troponin I	4–8 hours	12–16 hours	30–40 times normal
Myoglobin	2–4 hours	9–12 hrs	30–40 times normal

Fortunately, an astute medical student ordered a myoglobin level on this patient, and the result was elevated.

5. How does this information influence the determination of a diagnosis?

Myoglobin is found in all muscle tissue, including heart muscle. Injury to any muscle from sources as disparate as blunt trauma and chemical or metabolic disorders may release myoglobin into the bloodstream. Although it is nonspecific, an elevated serum myoglobin level is probably the best indicator of an MI within the first 6 hours of the onset of chest pain. This is especially true if there is no evidence to suggest a metabolic or physical insult prior to measuring the level. In this case, the myoglobin elevation in combination with this patient's history and ECG findings strongly suggest an acute MI as a diagnosis. It should be noted that this patient's chest pain initially occurred during her morning walk. Heart attacks frequently occur in the morning and during exercise. Platelets clump more readily in the morning, and exercise increases the demand for blood to the cardiac muscle.

ASSESSMENT

This patient has most likely suffered an **acute myocardial infarction**. The plan is to admit her to the cardiac care unit of the hospital and to arrange for a consult by a cardiologist.

6. What treatment options are available for this patient?

Discussion

The approach to the patient with an acute MI is complicated and controversial. Many physicians currently disagree about the best form of treatment. Options include thrombolytic therapy with agents such as streptokinase or cardiac catheterization with balloon angioplasty. After coronary angioplasty, stents can be inserted to diminish the chances of recurring stenosis. Different approaches to the coronary patient depend on the physician, the patient, and the individual circumstances. However, close observation is always necessary following ischemic events because patients are prone to arrhythmias that are potentially life-threatening.

CASE 5-2

INITIAL PRESENTATION

A 47-year-old woman complains of chest pain of 1-day duration. The pain is described as moderately severe, substernal in location, and radiating to her left shoulder. It is exacerbated by deep breathing and cough and is slightly relieved by sitting up. It is not relieved by resting and is unaffected by eating or drinking. The patient reports having had a temperature of 102.2°F. She has a 20-year history of scleroderma.

PHYSICAL EXAMINATION

The patient appears slightly flushed and acutely ill. Her vital signs are as follows: blood pressure, 122/88 mm Hg; pulse, 96 beats/min; and temperature, 102.2°F. The patient's respirations are rapid and shallow; her lungs are clear to percussion and auscultation. The patient's heart is beating at a regular rate. A fine friction rub is present during presystole, systole, and diastole. The remainder of the physical examination is unremarkable.

7. How might deep breathing, cough, and changing position affect chest pain?

Discussion

The signs and symptoms in this patient bear many similarities to those in Case 5-1. The most obvious is the presence of radiating substernal chest pain. In addition, the pain is acute. However, there are several notable differences, the most important being that this patient's pain is slightly positional and unrelated to activity. As discussed in the cases on abdominal pain (see Case 2-1), the organ parenchymal disorders often present with constant pain, whereas pathologies involving outer covering layers tend to be localized and may change with position (e.g., peritonitis). In the chest cavity, involvement of the pleura and the pericardium can cause positional pain. A deep breath pulls on the pericardium, and the pain from this inflamed structure may worsen. Changing position alters the location of the heart within the pericardial sac, and the pressure differences may affect the pain. Likewise, a cough may exert changing tensions on the pericardium. Fever in this patient indicates the presence of an infectious or inflammatory process.

The physical examination is very helpful in this case. As in the case of Mrs. M., the absence of lung findings helps exclude a pulmonary etiology. In this patient, however, there are some clearly localizing factors. The friction rub on cardiac auscultation is virtually pathognomonic for pericarditis. This diagnosis is supported by this patient's history of scleroderma. There is a variety of etiologies for acute pericarditis, including connective tissue disorders, as shown in Table 5-2.

LABORATORY TESTS

The patient's chest radiograph is within normal limits, although her heart appears slightly enlarged compared with a radiograph performed a few months ago. An ECG showed elevated ST segments in all leads except aVR and V_1. LDH, AST, and CK levels are mildly elevated.

8. Does the fact that the ECG has changes in most leads suggest widespread cardiac involvement?

TABLE 5-2
CAUSES OF ACUTE PERICARDITIS

Type of Etiology	Specific Disease or Disorder
Connective tissue disorders	Lupus erythematosus
	Rheumatoid arthritis
	Scleroderma
Infections	Viral infections
	Bacterial infections (including tuberculosis)
	Fungal (e.g., histoplasmosis)
Cancer	Metastatic lung cancer
	Metastatic breast cancer
	Lymphoma
Trauma	Blunt chest trauma
	Sharp wounds
	Internal rupture or aneurysm
Metabolic disorders	Uremia
	Myxedema
Iatrogenic	Surgical
	Radiation
	Hemodialysis
Drug-induced	Hydralazine
	Procainamide
	Niacin
Post-MI	
Idiopathic	

Discussion

Other historic information supporting the diagnosis of pericarditis is radiation of pain to the shoulder or commonly the trapezius muscle. The laboratory findings help confirm the diagnosis. Chest radiographs often are normal. The slightly enlarged heart, however, may indicate slight pericardial effusion. An echocardiogram may be helpful in this patient to determine the degree of effusion. Slight elevation in cardiac enzymes also may indicate that the outer portion of the myocardium is involved. Widespread ST-segment elevation is typical in patients with pericarditis. Occasionally, ST-segment depression is seen in the right-sided leads. Inflammation of the pericardium may spread to the epicardium, causing diffuse ST-segment changes. In summary, it is the positional nature of the pain and associated friction rub in this patient that help differentiate involvement of the pericardium from the myocardium as in Case 5-1.

ASSESSMENT

The acute onset, history of connective tissue disorder, and laboratory results help narrow the diagnosis to **acute pericarditis**. Anti-inflammatory treatment will be initiated (e.g., 900 mg aspirin, 3 or 4 times a day). The treatment plan for this patient includes an echocardiogram to evaluate the existence and degree of pericardial effusion. If the echocardiogram shows a large pericardial effusion, a cardiologist should follow the patient for possible tamponade, which can be fatal if untreated. Additional laboratory tests will be performed including viral titers, fungal and tuberculosis skin tests, and blood cultures. If these tests indicate a viral etiology, or at least the absence of fungus, bacteria, or tuberculosis, then bed rest and aspirin are the only treatments available. Full recovery is the norm. If the additional tests indicate bacteria, fungus, or tuberculosis as the etiologic agent, then a life-threatening condition exists, and an infectious disease specialist, as well as a cardiologist, should be involved in this patient's care. Complex regimens of parenteral and often multiple drugs may be necessary to effect a cure.

CASE 5-3

INITIAL PRESENTATION

A 66-year-old man complains of chest pain and shortness of breath for 2 days. His current problems began abruptly after a "cold" 2 days ago. He noted shaking chills and a cough productive of rust-colored sputum. The chest pain is right-sided, sharp, and much worse with deep breathing and coughing. The medical history is significant for chronic alcoholism and smoking.

PHYSICAL EXAMINATION

The patient appears acutely ill. His temperature is 104°F, and his breathing is rapid and shallow. A lung examination reveals that the right lower lobe has decreased breath sounds with some crackles in the periphery, dullness to percussion, and increased vocal fremitus. His cardiac examination is normal, as is the remainder of the physical examination.

9. What is the significance of shaking chills and rust-colored sputum?
10. How do the lung findings on physical examination influence the determination of a diagnosis?

Discussion

Similar to the situation in Case 5-2, it is worth noting that this patient's chest pain is positional and began acutely. Again, pain that is worse with movement often indicates involvement of a lining, such as the pericardium or pleura of the lung. The acute onset, chills, and high temperature are all consistent with an infectious process. The historical information about cough productive of sputum supports an infectious process, and involvement of the lungs and pink- or rust-colored sputum generally indicate the presence of red blood cells (RBCs). The physical examination helps confirm and further localize the diagnosis. The lung findings suggest right lower lobe consolidation consistent with pneumonia.

ASSESSMENT

This patient is diagnosed with **right lower lobe pneumonia**. His treatment plan includes performing a chest radiograph and obtaining sputum for Gram's stain, culture, and sensitivity. A complete blood cell count (CBC) with differential will be performed, and blood samples will be cultured. Antibiotic treatment will eventually be necessary depending on the Gram's stain result, but only after blood and sputum have been sent for culture.

The most common form of bacterial pneumonia is caused by *Streptococcus pneumoniae*. The disease often occurs following an upper respiratory viral infection and is much more common in patients older than 50 years, particularly if such individuals suffer from a chronic immunocompromising illness (e.g., diabetes, renal disease, alcoholism). Damage to respiratory epithelium due to chronic smoking is also a predisposing factor. There is considerable evidence that factors such as chronic illness and an acute insult (e.g., an upper respiratory infection) are directly involved in the pathogenesis of this disease because 5%–40% of healthy individuals carry *S. pneumoniae* in their nasopharynx. Unfortunately, this often may lead to complications when analyzing sputum for diagnosis. In this particular individual, however, if evidence of *S. pneumoniae* is found on Gram's stain of the sputum, penicillin treatment should be started prior to confirmation with cultures. If treatment is successful, this patient should be given a pneumococcal vaccine injection once he has recovered because of his high disposition for this type of pneumonia.

CASE 5-4

INITIAL PRESENTATION

A 55-year-old man complains of sudden onset of severe shortness of breath and left-sided chest pain. He is currently hospitalized and immobilized because of a recent motor vehicle accident. His pain is generally dull and diffuse on the left side, but becomes sharp and worse with movement and inspiration. There is an associated hemoptysis and cough. The patient expired before laboratory test results were obtained.

11. What anatomic involvement could cause dull chest pain that becomes sharp with movement and inspiration?

Discussion

The sudden onset of pain anywhere suggests a vascular or occlusive process. The dull chest pain may suggest involvement of organ parenchyma, whereas the sharper pain exacerbated by movement can indicate pleural involvement. The associated hemoptysis and cough further implicate lung involvement. Based on these factors, **pulmonary embolism** is the most likely diagnosis because blocking blood supply to an entire segment or lobe of a lung affects both the parenchyma and the pleura. Although ambulatory, healthy individuals may be affected, most pulmonary emboli occur in hospitalized or immobilized patients with a history of trauma or surgery. Being older than 50 years of age is also a significant risk factor. Although the clinical presentation is often variable, depending on the location and size of the emboli, this diagnosis should always be suspected in patients with these risk factors who present with sudden onset of dyspnea with or without chest pain. The clinical symptoms depend mainly on the number of emboli and the structures that are subsequently affected. Small emboli may result only in transient dyspnea. Multiple or larger emboli can result in more severe consequences, such as pulmonary infarction, pleural effusion, right-sided heart failure, and even complete cardiopulmonary failure. Most patients who succumb to an embolic event do so within the first few hours after onset.

ASSESSMENT

Currently, pulmonary embolism is one of the most common causes of preventable hospital deaths. Most often, the emboli originate from the deep veins in the leg. As a result, prevention of deep venous thrombosis (DVT) is important for prophylaxis of this disorder. High-risk patients may undergo Doppler studies if a DVT is suspected. In addition, close monitoring of the coagulation states of such a patient is recommended. Early ambulation following surgery or other medical procedures also prevents DVT formation. Finally, compression boots are often used on patients who are not ambulatory for long periods of time to prevent stasis.

CASE 5-5

INITIAL PRESENTATION

A 42-year-old man with Marfan syndrome presents to the emergency department complaining of abrupt onset of severe chest pain. He states that the pain began 2 hours ago and is "unbearable" and not relieved with pain control medications. The pain radiates to his left shoulder and jaw, it is constant, and is not relieved by resting. There is no change with movement. He has no history of hypertension, hypercholesterolemia, or diabetes.

PHYSICAL EXAMINATION

The patient appears acutely ill and in severe distress. His vital signs are: blood pressure, 104/68 mm Hg; pulse, 124 beats/min; and respirations, 22 breaths/min. His lungs are clear to percussion and auscultation. Cardiac examination reveals a rapid, regular heart beat. A soft holodiastolic murmur is heard loudest at the right border of the sternum at approximately the second intercostal space.

LABORATORY TESTS

An ECG shows sinus tachycardia but is otherwise unremarkable. A chest radiograph shows widening of the upper mediastinal shadow.

ASSESSMENT

This is another instance of sudden-onset chest pain, again suggesting a possible vascular process. The severe chest pain radiating to the jaw should raise concerns about a possible coronary event. However, there are some aspects of this case that differentiate it from Case 5-1. First, this patient's pain is constant and not relieved with rest. Second, he does not have the "typical" risk factors for coronary artery disease. Third, the murmur heard on physical examination suggests aortic valve regurgitation. It is important to note that there is no way of knowing whether this finding is acute without asking the patient or reviewing the medical record. Cardiac disease cannot be ruled out on the basis of this history. Widening of the mediastinum on the chest radiograph is a fairly nondescript finding, but it could help support an aortic arch or valve disorder. Lastly, the ECG tracing shows no signs of cardiac ischemia. If the tracing was done while the patient was still in pain, and the myocardium was involved, one would expect ST-segment changes.

As discussed previously, a quick review of the organs in the chest, as well as a basic understanding of clinical pathologic presentations, yields a probable diagnosis in this patient. The history suggests a circulatory or vascular event. In addition, the physical examination and chest radiograph show some evidence that the upper mediastinum and perhaps the aortic valve may be involved. The medical history of Marfan syndrome places this patient at risk for an ascending, dissecting aortic aneurysm. It is not uncommon for dissecting aortic aneurysms to present with pain similar to that of myocardial ischemia. Aneurysms involving the ascending limb of the aortic arch often radiate pain to the upper extremities and jaw, whereas those affecting the descending aorta tend to radiate pain to the abdomen or lower extremities. Transesophageal echocardiography usually confirms the diagnosis.

The diagnosis for this patient is **probable ascending dissecting aortic aneurysm**. His treatment plan involves transesophageal echocardiography and a thoracic surgical consult.

SUMMARY

There are several other causes of chest pain in addition to those presented in this chapter. Many can be diagnosed with a high degree of certainty using only the history, physical examination, and perhaps minimal testing (e.g., chest radiograph). For example, chest wall pain from fibromyalgia or intercostal muscle strain or tear are reproducible with movements or external pressure and are not usually confused with more life-threatening heart, lung, or vascular disorders. Herpes zoster involving the thoracic nerves occasionally may be puzzling, especially if the pain persists for several days before the characteristic rash appears.

The nature and associated characteristics of chest pain often provide invaluable clues for diagnosis. In addition, consideration of the relatively small number of organs within the thoracic cavity usually helps limit the potential diagnoses prior to laboratory investigation. However, the obvious initial concern with chest pain is a myocardial event; when myocardial ischemia is suspected, an ECG tracing and cardiac enzyme measurements should be performed. The diagnostic difficulties usually arise because cardiac disorders may present very similarly to gastrointestinal pathologies and vice versa. Any sudden-onset chest pain must be assumed to be potentially life-threatening because a functional compromise of any of the thoracic organs may result in the patient's immediate demise.

CHAPTER 6

Chief Complaint: Headache

CASE 6-1

INITIAL PRESENTATION

Ms. B., a 14-year-old girl, is brought to the clinic by her mother, who is worried about a headache her daughter has had for 2 days. The patient reports that she first noticed this headache upon waking up yesterday morning. Since then it has waxed and waned, but it has increased in intensity overall. She describes the headache as "throbbing" and localized to the right side. The headache is aggravated by bright light and loud noises. She has taken aspirin and acetaminophen, which have been only minimally effective. The patient also has associated nausea and vomiting, which gets worse as the headache becomes more intense. She describes the pain as a six or seven on a scale of one to ten. Although she has never experienced a headache that has lasted this long, she does admit to severe headaches in the past. The patient denies previous head trauma and states that she noted no symptoms prior to the onset of the headache. She takes no medications on a regular basis. Although the patient notes no change, her mother reports that she "has not been herself" for the last 3 days. The mother tells you that the night prior to the onset of her headache, Ms. B. seemed depressed, which was unusual for her. Ms. B. was adopted, so, unfortunately, a family history is unavailable.

1. What is the mechanism resulting in headache?
2. What is the significance of localized pain?
3. Why is a medication history important in this case?
4. Why might a family history be helpful in this case?

Discussion

Headache occurs with stimulation of pain-sensitive nerves in structures such as parts of the dura mater, the basilar arteries, the sensory cranial nerves, and extracranial tissues (e.g., skin). The brain itself cannot sense pain; however, it can interpret certain sensory input as headache. Pathologies and symptomatology in the head are different from other regions of the body because the head consists of very soft tissues almost completely enclosed by bone.

The sensation of pain can be experienced only when structures that are innervated by sensory neurons are involved. Generalized pain occurs when a pathologic process involves relatively poorly innervated structures or causes diffuse involvement. Localized pain, on the other hand, results from isolated effects on richly innervated tissues. The word "effects" is important because a pathologic process may or may not actually be occurring within the sensory structure to cause pain. Mass lesions, such as tumors, cause pain by stretching or pushing on nerves that are often in a remote location of the cranium. As a general rule, pain from mass lesions localize to the side with the lesion. For example, masses in the right occipital region often result in right-sided pain, but the headache may be felt in the right parietal or occipital regions.

A medication history is always important for ruling out a drug reaction or interaction problem, and it can sometimes lead to a very quick diagnosis and treatment plan. A variety of medications such as trimethoprim/sulfamethoxazole, nitrates, and antihypertensive agents can cause headache.

Tension headaches and migraines tend to run in families. Thus, a positive family history in association with pertinent signs and symptoms may strongly indicate one of these conditions.

PHYSICAL EXAMINATION

Her head is examined for any anomalies or signs of trauma, and her ears, nose, and throat (ENT) are examined for signs of sinusitis or allergy. A thorough physical examination proves unremarkable.

5. What are the most important physical examination maneuvers to perform on a patient with a headache?
6. With a physical examination that is unremarkable, what should be done next?

Discussion

Of particular importance is a good head, ears, eyes, nose, and throat (HEENT) examination. An ophthalmologic examination can be particularly helpful if one has reason to suspect the patient might have increased intracranial pressure. In such a case, one should look closely for papilledema. A complete ENT examination also can be quite valuable because pathology in any of these areas can cause headache. In particular, an ENT examination should be directed toward any signs of sinusitis or allergy, as these are two of the most common causes of headache. In addition, dental disorders are notorious for causing headaches. Visual acuity also should be evaluated to rule out orbital or retro-orbital involvement, although, despite the common belief, vision problems account for fewer than 2% of headaches. For obvious reasons, a thorough neurologic examination, including mental status, should be conducted on any individual if a cause for a headache is not readily apparent after taking the history. A headache, serious or not, often involves a pathology that affects a portion of the head or neck. As a result, a variety of headache disorders can affect neurologic function.

In any patient with a headache, the initial diagnostic steps should always be directed toward ruling out a life-threatening cause. Fortunately, this often can be accomplished via a thorough history and physical. Ms. B.'s headache, although obviously disturbing, is not the worst she has ever experienced. In addition, the symptoms did not begin suddenly, as they might with a vascular problem. The lack of associated neurologic symptoms, physical examination findings, or history of trauma, all make a life-threatening pathology much less likely. Head-imaging studies, such as a computerized tomography (CT) scan or magnetic resonance imaging (MRI) scan, as well as a lumbar puncture (LP), might be considered in a patient in whom an intracranial lesion, a hemorrhage, or meningeal abnormality is suspected. However, a young person with a unilateral, throbbing headache that is aggravated by light and sound is very likely suffering from a common migraine headache. These headaches are, as the name suggests, much more prevalent than classic migraines, which are preceded by an aura. Many patients also note visual disturbances. Migraines tend to run in families, they are more common in women, and they are often associated with nausea and vomiting. Many patients suffer from migraines for many years, and others may have only one episode. Those with frequent attacks often identify initiating factors, such as certain foods, drugs, changes in sleep pattern, or menstrual cycle.

7. What medications could be given to Ms. B. to treat her migraine headache?

Several medications have proven helpful in the treatment of migraine headaches, although many patients suffer from debilitating attacks that are not significantly relieved by pharmacologic intervention. The classic treatment for migraine has been ergotamine, although this is usually only effective when begun very early in the attack. In those patients who have a noticeable prodrome, such as altered vision, hearing, taste, or smell due to cerebrovascular constriction, ergotamine may prevent or greatly reduce the pain. Once the headache has begun, ergotamine is much less effective. Phenothiazines are effective in treating any associated nausea and, for unknown reasons, may also relieve the headache. In resistant or severe cases, narcotics may be necessary.

More recently, sumatriptan has become available as another effective agent to treat the acute pain of a migraine headache. Several medications, including β-blockers and tricyclic antidepressants, may reduce the frequency of migraines when taken on a regular basis.

ASSESSMENT

Ms. B. is diagnosed with **common migraine headache**. She is given intravenous phenothiazine in the emergency department, and her nausea and pain improve significantly during the next few hours until all symptoms resolve. She should be cautioned that recurrence of such headaches is quite possible. The patient should be asked to keep a diary of events if migraines persist, and follow-up should be performed in a clinic.

CASE 6-2

INITIAL PRESENTATION

A 77-year-old man is brought to the emergency department for a severe headache that began abruptly yesterday afternoon. The patient states that the headache is the worst he has ever had and describes the pain as diffuse and constant in nature. His wife reports that the patient has been forgetful and depressed since the onset of the headache. There are no identifiable precipitating, aggravating, or alleviating factors.

PHYSICAL EXAMINATION

The patient's vital signs are: blood pressure, 150/94 mm Hg; pulse, 96 beats/min; and temperature, 100.1°F. Nuchal rigidity is present; there are no focal neurologic deficits.

8. Does the sudden onset of the headache suggest a cause?
9. Is nuchal rigidity worrisome, and what may cause this sign?
10. What does the fever indicate?

Discussion

This case presentation is notably different from Case 6-1. Probably the most significant factors are the severity and abrupt onset of this patient's symptoms. Most headaches worked up in the emergency department setting do not involve serious intracranial disorders. Causes in patients who present with headache usually include migraines, tension, and sinusitis. Subarachnoid hemorrhage is a relatively uncommon cause of headache and is extremely rare in patients younger than 35 years. However, because of the seriousness of the disorder, it should be considered in any patient with sudden onset of severe head pain. Hemorrhage may be caused by factors such as trauma, intracranial aneurysm, arteriovenous malformation, leukemia, cerebral tumors, bleeding disorders, or anticoagulant therapy. Of these, rupture of a congenital aneurysm is the most common in the absence of known trauma to the head. In many cases, an initial bleed occurs hours to days before rupture of the aneurysm, and it may cause headache and other symptoms but no signs of an intracranial catastrophe until a vessel rupture occurs. The finding of nuchal rigidity suggests meningeal irritation, which often occurs in patients suffering from a subarachnoid hemorrhage. Focal neurologic deficits may or may not occur, depending on the size and location of the lesion. More generalized neurologic symptoms, such as confusion or alteration in mood, are common. Low-grade fever may occur with meningeal inflammation from any cause, including blood contact, and does not necessarily indicate infection.

11. What diagnostic steps might further delineate the problem?

Due to the strong suspicion of a vascular anomaly, a CT brain scan would be a reasonable next step for this patient. CT scans are diagnostic in almost 90% of subarachnoid hemorrhages, and they are helpful in determining prognosis and appropriate surgical intervention. If the scan is negative, a LP would confirm the diagnosis if elevated intracranial pressure and blood were present. Additionally, the LP may reveal other causes of meningeal irritation if a subarachnoid hemorrhage is not the culprit. Viral, bacterial, or fungal infections of the central nervous system (CNS) are possible but unlikely given the abrupt onset with no prodrome of other systemic symptoms. As soon as patients can be stabilized, angiography and surgical intervention are usually recommended.

ASSESSMENT

The history and physical examination of this patient yield evidence of meningeal irritation and an intracranial vascular event consistent with a **subarachnoid hemorrhage**. The management plan is to perform a CT scan and to arrange for a neurosurgical consult.

Unfortunately, prognosis for a full recovery is not good for most patients with a subarachnoid hemorrhage. Long-term consequences among survivors range from permanent, localized, neurologic defects to coma. In addition, subsequent rebleeding and cerebral ischemia secondary to vascular spasm are not uncommon. Although supportive care, pharmacologic intervention, and some surgical procedures are usually helpful, the morbidity and mortality in patients with subarachnoid hemorrhage are unfortunately quite high. Recent advancements in rehabilitation techniques have lessened the long-term functional deficits of these patients.

CASE 6-3

INITIAL PRESENTATION

A 24-year-old medical student comes to the clinic complaining of a headache that he describes as "dull and pressing" in a band-like pattern. He says the pain is "mild" but disturbing because it has occurred on a daily basis for the past several months. The patient reports that it is usually worse at the end of the day and is helped slightly by aspirin. There are no associated neurologic or other symptoms. The patient states that his mother also has headaches "all the time."

12. Do the signs and symptoms suggest serious intracranial pathology?

Discussion

The band-like pattern is classic for tension headaches. Most tension headaches are relatively mild and are described by patients as dull or pressing. They often run in families and are usually helped to some degree by over-the-counter analgesics. As in the case of Ms. B. (Case 6-1), the absence of associated neurologic or other symptoms helps rule out a more serious or localized cause of this patient's problem.

PHYSICAL EXAMINATION

The physical examination is within normal limits.

13. What is the pathogenesis of tension headaches?

Discussion

The answer to this question is not as straightforward as one might think. Pericranial muscle contraction is clearly associated with the disorder, but "the chicken or the egg" debate has recently become an issue. It was previously thought these headaches were the result of painful, chronic contraction of the muscles of the scalp and neck as a result of fatigue or stress. However, some experts now suspect that tension headaches may have the same underlying pathologic process as vascular headaches, such as seen in Ms. B. (Case 6-1). Therefore, pericranial muscle contraction would be the result rather than the cause of the headache. The severity of tension headaches varies. Most people occasionally experience headache in stressful situations. Some suffer from headaches more often and also have trouble dealing with stress on a constant basis. The extreme end of the spectrum involves patients who suffer from dull, chronic headaches on a constant basis and who may experience more severe headaches with an apparent vascular component.

14. How should this patient's case be managed?

Whether there is a common pathology involved in tension headaches and migraines, it is clear that tension headaches are partly the result of stress, fatigue, or a combination of both. Furthermore, these are the most common types of headaches reported to physicians. In mild cases, treatment is often straightforward, involving stress relief, avoidance of fatigue, and minimal use of over-the-counter analgesics. The diagnosis is usually fairly clear from the history and physical; response to therapy is good, although headaches may recur. More severe cases, however, may present more of a problem. In some cases, a CT scan of the brain or an LP may actually be required, if only to reassure the patient that no serious, life-threatening process is involved. In addition, chronic use of analgesics can be problematic. Regular use of aspirin and other nonsteroidal anti-inflammatory drugs (NSAIDs) may cause stomach irritation and even ulcers. Paradoxically, prolonged use of analgesics may actually worsen the pain in some patients. Patient dependence on both narcotic and non-narcotic analgesics may develop. There is a small group of patients in whom severe headaches occur on a daily basis and are not relieved by anything. These patients can be extremely difficult to manage, as they often place extraordinary demands on their physicians. Referral to a pain clinic or headache specialist may be the best plan for these individuals.

ASSESSMENT

The medical student is suffering from **tension headaches**. The treatment plan for this patient consists of stress relief and rest. Aspirin or acetaminophen may be used sparingly when needed.

CASE 6-4

INITIAL PRESENTATION

A 52-year-old man presents complaining of a severe headache that began in the left frontal area but is now more diffuse. It began insidiously 3–4 weeks ago and is progressively getting worse. The patient describes the pain as "severe" and different from headaches he has had before. He states that the pain is constant, but slightly worse in the morning. His wife reports that he has been increasingly forgetful and irritable during the past few months but lately just seems "depressed." The patient's history includes a lung neoplasm removed surgically 2 years ago and subsequently treated with chemotherapy.

PHYSICAL EXAMINATION

The patient's vital signs are within normal limits. Papilledema is noted; otherwise his HEENT examination is normal. There are no focal neurologic deficits; his cranial nerves are intact.

15. Does the insidious onset and progressive change in the nature of the pain direct the thought process in forming a diagnosis?
16. Is papilledema a minor or major finding?

Discussion

Compared with Ms. B. in Case 6-1, there are several differences in this patient's presentation that cause concern. One worry is that this is a new type of headache for this patient. As illustrated in the previous case, headaches are common, and many individuals suffer from headaches routinely. However, a new type of headache, especially one that is severe, suggests a pathologic process that the patient has not previously experienced. Another worrisome aspect of this patient's headache is that it is worsening, and this implies that the condition might be progressive. Also, the headache was initially localized but is now generalized, possibly indicating that the pathologic process involved is now having a global affect. Headaches caused by increased intracranial pressure are often worse in the morning and are exacerbated by coughing or straining. Therefore, it is possible that an initially localized abnormality has progressed and is now causing increased pressure by occluding the flow of cerebrospinal fluid (CSF). The change in recent mood and cognition could also suggest that neural tissue is being affected, although this is a somewhat "soft sign," because many individuals experience such changes with almost any illness. The finding of papilledema, however, is anything but a soft sign. It confirms the hypothesis of increased intracranial pressure and must be pursued.

All of these findings suggest a worsening pathologic process involving neural tissue. When these findings are analyzed in view of this patient's medical history, a metastatic cerebral neoplasm would be a primary concern. Brain tumors are generally independent of age and sex; therefore, they are one of the most common types of cancer in children. In adults, tumors may present as primary but are usually the result of metastasis from other tumors, such as those of the lung. It is common for intracranial masses to cause headaches that are worse when a patient first wakes up in the morning. In addition, growing masses may cause focal pain initially by stretching or pushing on local structures, but the pain gradually becomes generalized as more remote structures become involved with increasing intracranial pressure.

17. What should be done now toward making a diagnosis?

Intracranial masses cause associated symptoms in a variety of ways. Some tumors infiltrate and actually replace normal tissue. In addition, tumors may interfere with the flow of the CSF, causing increased intracranial pressure. Tumors also can physically displace normal tissue within the relatively unforgiving space of the skull. As a result, brain tumors may cause a variety of symptoms; although headache is the primary symptom in almost half of all cases, most cerebral neoplasms eventually result in other neurologic problems. In general, a headache is more indicative of tumor when it is associated with other symptoms, when it is a new type for a patient who does not normally complain of headaches, or when it represents a change in a chronic headache disorder. The most common symptom of an intracranial mass is a new-onset seizure. However, for the reasons discussed above, virtually any neurologic deficit may accompany this disorder, depending on the area of the brain affected. Also, the region of the brain causing signs and symptoms may be remote from the site of the lesion but induce compression of the affected area against the skull or other structures.

ASSESSMENT

There is **increased intracranial pressure** in this patient, who has a history of a cancer that frequently metastasizes to the brain.

Few laboratory tests are effective in diagnosing intracranial neoplasms. CT scans may detect some lesions, particularly if a tumor is large enough to displace brain tissue significantly. However, an MRI with contrast is much more helpful because this imaging technique is more sensitive than a CT and can help determine if the blood–brain barrier has been compromised. The physician orders an oncology consult and an MRI of the brain.

CASE 6-5

INITIAL PRESENTATION

A 44-year-old man complains of a series of severe headaches that began when he was in his early thirties and have now become more severe. The patient states that the headaches often awaken him from sleep. He describes them as usually beginning as a dull ache behind the left eye then rapidly spreading to severe pain in the temporal area and on the left side of his face. There is associated tearing of the left eye and facial flushing. The patient's headaches usually last 2–3 hours and occur several times a day for several days and then do not recur for 3–4 months. There are no associated neurologic symptoms. The patient has had two CT scans and an MRI, both of which were normal.

PHYSICAL EXAMINATION

The physical examination is unremarkable. The patient is symptom free at the time.

18. What pathophysiologic mechanism could cause unilateral pain that is episodic and not associated with an abnormal brain scan?

Discussion

This case is reminiscent of Ms. B. (Case 6-1) in that there is severe headache confined to one side. Thus, a localized process is likely. In addition, the absence of neurologic symptoms and the normal physical examination help rule out a pathology affecting neurologic function. Severe worsening pain is always a concern. Fortunately, this patient's condition is chronic and generally stable. As a result, a serious life-threatening disorder (e.g., tumor, vascular disorder) is highly unlikely; the normal CT and MRI scans obviously help to eliminate such disorders. Whatever is occurring in this patient is clearly periodic. Tension headaches do not usually present on one side, and they do not fit an episodic pattern as seen here. Nor do they cause the associated tearing and facial flushing. However, a vasodilatation condition, as seen in Case 6-1, is a distinct possibility. Such a disorder would be localized, intermittent, and would not show findings on imaging studies. This pattern is a classic presentation of cluster headaches, a disorder that involves a vasodilating pathology, is much less common than migraine, and, as the name suggests, occurs in clusters interrupted by long periods when the patient is asymptomatic. The disorder is more common in men, generally presents in the third to fourth decade, and typically worsens as the patient ages. Lacrimation and rhinorrhea are common, and they indicate trigeminoparasympathetic involvement.

19. What treatment is appropriate for this patient?

The initial pharmacologic treatments for cluster headaches are, not surprisingly, similar to those used for migraines. Usual therapy includes preventive agents such as calcium channel blockers, β-blockers, and even lithium or prednisone. Drugs to abort an attack include sumatriptan, ergot alkaloids, and narcotics. Less well-established treatments include melatonin, streptomycin-lidocaine injections, and magnesium sulfate. The variety of drug types may indicate multiple causes of cluster headaches. Surgical intervention to ablate trigeminal sensory fibers is occasionally necessary in patients who do not respond to drug treatment. This patient is given a prescription for verapamil. The effectiveness of the medication and his condition will be followed up in a clinic.

ASSESSMENT

This patient is diagnosed with **cluster headaches**. Although the history is usually all that is required for diagnosis, many patients undergo numerous investigative studies and failed treatment plans prior to diagnosis. Whether the physician is aware of the pattern of cluster headaches, the most important diagnostic reasoning strategy is that discussed above: The localized, episodic pattern, coupled with a lack of findings on CT or MRI scans strongly suggests some sort of vascular phenomenon.

CASE 6-6

INITIAL PRESENTATION

A 23-year-old woman complains of a frontal headache that has lasted for 2 days. She has had headaches similar to this in the past but none this severe. The headaches usually occur at the same time each year, and they are associated with nasal congestion and rhinorrhea, which the patient attributes to seasonal allergies that she has suffered since she was a child. There are no associated neurologic symptoms.

PHYSICAL EXAMINATION

The patient's vital signs are normal. There is tenderness to light tapping over the frontal and maxillary areas. The ophthalmologic examination is normal. There are no focal or generalized neurologic deficits. The remainder of the physical examination is normal.

20. What is the leading hypothesis at this time?

Discussion

Although this headache is more severe than any the patient has experienced in the past, this condition is obviously chronic and recurrent. As with Cases 6-1, 6-3, and 6-5, the absence of associated neurologic and ophthalmologic findings makes a potentially life-threatening disorder less likely. Furthermore, the history and physical examination suggest a localized process. The annual occurrence, seasonal allergies, nasal congestion, and rhinorrhea are probably the most important historic aspects of this case. Allergies may lead to infection, which unfortunately can cause even more allergy problems. This patient most likely suffers from seasonal allergies that are now exacerbated by a sinus infection. Tenderness to tapping on the maxillary and frontal sinuses suggests inflammation in adjacent tissues. Although a CT scan may be useful to diagnose patients refractory to treatment, antibiotics and decongestant therapy often are implemented prior to definitive diagnosis. An antihistamine and a nasal steroid also might be used to address the allergic component.

ASSESSMENT

This patient is suffering from **seasonal allergies exacerbated by sinusitis**. Her treatment plan includes a decongestant (e.g., astemizole) and an antibiotic (e.g., amoxicillin). Nasal steroids and an antihistamine can be taken as needed for allergies.

CASE 6-7

INITIAL PRESENTATION

An 83-year-old woman complains of worsening headaches during the past 3 months. The headaches begin as an intermittent burning sensation over her right temple. She now describes it as "constant" and "sore." There are associated fevers, body aches, and malaise.

PHYSICAL EXAMINATION

The woman's temperature is 102.4°F. She appears ill and in moderate distress. Examination of her head reveals a prominent right temporal artery. The area around the artery is erythematous and tender to the touch.

LABORATORY TESTS

Her erythrocyte sedimentation rate (ESR) is markedly increased at 110 mm/hr.

21. What is the importance of the tenderness and erythema?
22. Do the fever, body aches, and malaise suggest systemic involvement?

Discussion

This case clearly is different from the others in this chapter in that an extracranial process is at least partly involved. It is noteworthy that this patient describes more of a "sore" feeling than a true headache. In addition, the physical examination is consistent with a superficial inflammatory process. ESR is a nonspecific test but is generally a sensitive measure of inflammation or necrosis. Although biopsy would be necessary for definitive diagnosis, evidence of an inflamed temporal artery suggests, not surprisingly, temporal arteritis. The finding of erythema is quite helpful in this patient, but not absolutely necessary for diagnosis. In most cases, the affected area is not erythematous. The disease is common among elderly patients but extremely rare in individuals younger than 30 years. Women have the disease far more often than men.

23. What is the pathology of temporal arteritis?
24. What is an appropriate treatment plan?

Temporal arteritis is a granulomatous inflammation of the medium and small arteries, typically involving cranial vessels. The local findings may be part of a much more widespread giant cell arteritis, and it is, therefore, common for patients to suffer from more generalized symptoms also, such as fever, weight loss, fatigue, arthralgias, and malaise. The exact cause of this disorder is still a mystery, but probably involves some type of cell-mediated immunity against antigens in the arterial wall. Some familial clustering occurs, and a genetic component is suspected.

Temporal arteritis can be quite serious if left untreated because, in addition to the superficial arteries of the scalp, other crucial vessels such as those of the eye and, in some cases, the brain may be affected. Roughly half of the patients develop some degree of blindness from retinal artery occlusion if the disease is left untreated. Fortunately, the disease is quite responsive to corticosteroid therapy, which reduces inflammation, alleviates symptoms, and dramatically lowers the incidence of arterial occlusion. The ESR drops quickly and is used to monitor the dose of corticosteroid and length of treatment time. Unfortunately, therapy is usually required for months or even years. Because long-term steroid therapy has potential serious complications, it is important to use the lowest effective dose and to switch to an every-other-day regimen as soon as possible. Methods to prevent steroid osteoporosis also should be instituted, especially in older women who are prone to this condition. Because the treatment is prolonged and risky, a temporal artery biopsy to confirm giant cell arteritis should be done immediately upon suspecting the diagnosis. Some loss of vision may occur quickly, so the relatively benign biopsy procedure should be scheduled promptly. More than 48 hours of corticosteroid therapy may invalidate histologic confirmation.

ASSESSMENT

This patient is diagnosed with **temporal arteritis** and is suspected of being affected with giant cell arteritis. The patient is scheduled for an immediate temporal artery biopsy. Steroid treatment is started, and close follow-up with regular ESR measurements is scheduled. Measures to minimize the side effects of corticosteroids (e.g., osteoporosis) are instituted.

SUMMARY

Headaches are one of the most common patient complaints. They may be associated with a variety of disorders that range from benign to immediately life-threatening. An appropriate history and physical examination (focused on the timing, pattern, intensity, location, and associated symptoms or deficits) are the most important steps toward diagnosis. Of particular importance in the diagnostic process is timing or onset and any associated neurologic deficits.

CHAPTER 7

Chief Complaint: Dizziness

CASE 7-1

INITIAL PRESENTATION

Mr. J., a 56-year-old plumber, presents with a complaint of feeling "dizzy." Upon further questioning, the patient states that "it feels like the room is spinning around." The episodes have occurred three times in the past week. They usually begin fairly suddenly when he changes position, such as when he bends down to tie his shoe or pick up pipes at work. He has never actually fallen down, but he feels like he could easily do so. Mr. J. states that when the episodes occur he sits down for a few minutes and then feels fine. At first, he thought that these "attacks" would just go away, but now he is concerned that they might indicate something worse.

> Indication of vertigo

> Trigger

The patient denies any other associated symptoms, such as tinnitus, hearing loss, headaches, paresthesias, ataxia, episodes of incoordination, visual disturbances, speech difficulties, and changes of consciousness. The patient's medical history is largely unremarkable. Mr. J. denies any previous psychiatric disorders as well as any symptoms of anxiety or depression. He suffers from no chronic illnesses and takes no medications on a regular basis.

> The associated signs and symptoms are a key in differentiating central dizziness from a vestibular disorder.

> Other possible causes of dizziness

1. What information is needed to determine what this patient means by "dizzy"?
2. How is balance normally controlled?
3. Why is a medication history particularly important in this case?

Discussion

Patients may describe a variety of different symptoms as "dizzy" spells. Unfortunately, the word "dizzy" is fairly nondescript; therefore, it is important to differentiate whether a patient is referring to orthostatic lightheadedness or vertigo.

Balance is controlled via input to the central nervous system (CNS) from several systems. The systems are slightly redundant, so that the loss of one would not prohibit an individual from standing or walking. However, malfunction of any one of these systems or of the connections between them can cause dizziness. The visual system uses light stimuli to relay data about head position relative to the horizontal. The proprioceptive system uses pressure stimuli from the peripheral nerves to relay data about the position and movement of the limbs. The peripheral vestibular system consists of the semicircular canals, the saccule, and the utricle in the inner ear. Cells in each of these structures have stereocilia stretching into the gelatinous perilymphatic fluid of the inner ear. Movement of the stereocilia results in signals to the CNS via the eighth cranial nerve (CN VIII). The semicircular canals provide information about angular movement of the head, whereas the utricle and saccule provide information about acceleration of the head and its relationship to gravity. Specifically, CN VIII relays this information to the vestibular nuclei in the brain stem. The vestibulo-ocular system also controls positioning of the eyes during head movement. (For example, you should be able to move your head from side to side while continuing to view this page.) Disturbances of the vestibulo-ocular system can result in abnormal movements of the eyes, known as nystagmus. The medulla, pons, and midline cerebellar structures coordinate and integrate information from each of these systems. Once a patient is determined to be suffering from vertigo, possible dysfunctions of any one of these structures or systems must be considered.

There are many medications that can cause dizziness by affecting primarily the vestibular system or the CNS. For example, aminoglycoside antibiotics (e.g., gentamicin) often affect the vestibular system. A variety of sedatives and antidepressants also are known to result in dizziness via their effects on the CNS. A medication history including prescriptions, over-the-counter drugs, and herbal remedies is always an important aspect of a medical history.

PHYSICAL EXAMINATION

Mr. J. appears to be a healthy, well-developed man in no apparent distress. His vital signs are: temperature, 98.2°F; pulse, 76 beats/

min; and blood pressure, 122/76 mm Hg. His extraocular movements (EOMs) are intact, and his vision is 20/20 bilaterally. Funduscopic examination is normal. Mr. J.'s hearing is good to a whispered voice. His tympanic membranes appear clear with good light reflex and no evidence of bulging or edema. Neurologically, Mr. J. is oriented to person, place, and time. His strength and sensation are normal in all extremities. CN II–XII are intact. Proprioception is normal, and cerebellar functions are intact. Mr. J. displays a normal gait. Romberg's test is normal; however, the head positioning maneuvers resulted in vertigo and nystagmus, which resolved within 1 minute.

4. Do the symptoms and signs point toward a CNS problem or a peripheral problem?

Discussion

In any patient with true vertigo, a complete history and physical examination focusing on neurologic diseases are very important. A variety of potentially serious CNS pathologies such as tumors or vascular accidents must be ruled out initially. In this case, the absence of such factors makes a peripheral disorder (e.g., inner ear or position sense) much more likely. However, there are few signs that might indicate an inner ear disturbance or other sensory pathologies. One potentially important aspect of Mr. J.'s symptoms is that they occur with sudden changes in position. This fact is confirmed by the positive head positioning maneuver, which indicates a vestibular dysfunction dependent on position. Various maneuvers are performed to diagnose vestibular dysfunction, but most involve head movement with one ear down and then with the other ear down. If the vertigo is reproduced, then the diagnosis of vestibular dysfunction is likely, and the problem is in the ear that was down when the symptoms occurred.

The most common cause of a peripheral disorder is benign positional vertigo (BPV), which is sometimes referred to as benign paroxysmal positional vertigo. BPV is the most common cause of vertigo. Fortunately, as the name implies, it is a relatively harmless disorder. However, as previously mentioned, it is extremely important to rule out other more dangerous etiologies before arriving at the diagnosis of BPV. Although the definitive cause of BPV remains somewhat of a mystery, the disorder is most likely caused by mineral deposits within the semicircular canals, which bend the hair cells in an abnormal fashion.

ASSESSMENT

5. What should the physician tell Mr. J. about his problem?
6. How might the physician afford Mr. J. some relief?

Discussion

Mr. J. is diagnosed with **BPV**. In some cases, BPV resolves spontaneously. If not, there are a variety of exercises, known as particle repositioning, which have proven successful in dislodging the deposits in the semicircular canals. Mr. J.'s treatment plan includes being scheduled for an instructional session to learn particle repositioning exercises. In other patients, pharmacologic and surgical intervention may be necessary. In any event, Mr. J. should be cautioned that the vertigo may strike without warning and that he should avoid situations where loss of balance might result in serious injury. Holding on to something or sitting down on the floor or ground until the episode resolves is prudent advice.

CASE 7-2

INITIAL PRESENTATION

A 77-year-old man complains of dizziness, and he describes "room spinning." His symptoms have not changed since they began suddenly 2 hours ago. The patient has associated numbness around his mouth as well as difficulty swallowing. He has a dull posterior headache and a history of hypertension.

PHYSICAL EXAMINATION

The patient is oriented but in obvious distress. His vital signs are: blood pressure, 160/110 mm Hg; pulse, 88 beats/min; and temperature, 100°F. Nystagmus is present, and it is independent of position. Perioral hyperesthesia is confirmed with pinprick testing. There are no carotid bruits.

7. How is this patient different from Mr. J. in Case 7-1?
8. How do these differences change the diagnostic possibilities for this patient?

Discussion

As in Case 7-1, it is important to differentiate between a peripheral and a central cause of vertigo. This case has some notable differences from Case 7-1. Although both patients are suffering from symptoms of vertigo, this patient's symptoms are unchanged by position. In addition, this patient has associated symptoms. The presence of nystagmus indicates that the vestibulo-ocular system is involved. Headache, particularly between the ears or in the back of the head, can result from either ear or brain pathology. Localized pain, such as behind the eye or in the forehead, may be indicative of brain disease. In this case, the constant nature of the vertigo, the headache, the perioral numbness, and the associated dysphagia are highly suggestive of a central cause of dizziness, such as a disturbance in the brain stem. There are a variety of CNS disorders that can potentially result in vertigo, but the sudden onset of this patient's symptoms make a vascular event likely. The patient's history of high blood pressure also is consistent with this diagnosis. Hypertension is the most common predisposing factor of stroke. An imaging study such as a computed tomography (CT) scan is necessary to confirm the diagnosis of a cerebrovascular event.

ASSESSMENT

This patient is suffering from **sudden-onset vertigo and headache**. He requires a CT scan to rule out stroke, and thrombolytic therapy should be considered.

CASE 7-3

INITIAL PRESENTATION

A 44-year-old woman complains of feeling "dizzy" for the past 2 weeks. With specific questioning, she describes episodes of being very lightheaded, like she is going to "pass out." She has never actually lost consciousness. Episodes occur when she moves from a sitting to a standing position or when she sits up quickly in bed. She has a history of chronic, poorly controlled hypertension despite treatment with a variety of antihypertensive medications. She was recently placed on prazosin for blood pressure control, and the lightheadedness began after this medication was initiated.

9. What is the leading hypothesis at this point?

Discussion

Although this patient is complaining of feeling "dizzy," she actually has a different complaint than the patients in Cases 7-1 and 7-2. This individual is having episodes of lightheadedness, not vertigo. The feeling of lightheadedness often is an indication that the brain is not being well perfused. A variety of disorders can result in poor cerebral perfusion, but the history often gives clues about the pathology. A transient ischemic attack (TIA), for example, causes decreased perfusion because microthromboemboli from peripheral sites such as the external carotid artery block cerebral blood vessels. These episodes are transient because the microthromboemboli are quickly broken up by thrombolytic factors. However, in this case, as in Case 7-1, the positional nature of the disorder may be a major clue. Besides occlusion of an artery, relative hypovolemia also can result in lightheadedness. There is no evidence of significant dehydration or blood loss in this patient, which means that the volume of blood may be normal but that it is not redistributed properly with sudden changes in position. In this particular patient, antihypertensive medication should be considered as a very likely cause of her "dizzy" spells because initiation of the drug is temporally related to the onset of the problem, and the medicine is known to work by dilating arterioles.

10. How is blood pressure normally regulated when moving from a supine to a standing position?

The blood vessels of the body essentially form a closed-loop circuit from the heart to the periphery and back to the heart again. As a result, blood leaving one area must be replaced by blood from another. However, blood vessels are distensible tubes that can be stretched and collapsed. When an individual stands up from a sitting position or sits up from a recumbent position, the vessels in the lower extremities expand because of the static weight of the blood above those vessels. These expanded veins (and to a lesser extent arteries) have a larger volume capacity and therefore can hold more blood. Because the vascular system is a closed loop, the larger volume of blood in the lower extremities, below the heart, results in (and is a result of) relatively less blood above the heart. The vessels that are located higher than the level of the heart tend to collapse because of the relatively lower pressure within the lumen of these vessels. For obvious reasons, however, the brain must remain fully perfused. Therefore, in normally functioning individuals, baroreceptors in the carotid arteries and aortic arch sense this drop in intraluminal pressure. The baroreceptors are merely stretch receptors. As the volume of blood in the aorta and the carotid arteries decreases, the walls of these vessels become less distended. This stimulus, in turn, causes a decrease in vagal tone and an increase in sympathetic tone throughout the body. As a result, the heart rate increases, shifting more blood from the venous to the arterial system, and peripheral vessels constrict. This increases total peripheral resistance and shunts blood to the brain.

PHYSICAL EXAMINATION

When supine, the patient's vital signs are: blood pressure, 148/96 mm Hg; and pulse, 82 beats/min. When standing, her vital signs are: blood pressure, 112/74 mm Hg; and pulse, 116 beats/min, with a subjective feeling of lightheadedness after 20 seconds. A neck examination reveals no carotid bruits. Her lungs are clear to percussion and auscultation. A cardiac examination indicates a regular rate without murmurs, gallops, or rubs. In her extremities, all peripheral pulses are 2+ bilaterally, with no peripheral edema. The remainder of the physical examination is unremarkable.

11. What might explain the drop in blood pressure upon standing?

Discussion

Although the positional characteristics of this patient's symptoms do not support a TIA as a cause of her lightheadedness, auscultation for carotid bruits is easy to do and is reasonable in this patient. The presence of carotid bruits could indicate a disturbance of blood flow consistent with a thrombus, which could throw off emboli. Although not at all conclusive, a normal cardiac examination helps ensure that the heart is functioning properly. The normal peripheral pulses are further indication that peripheral circulation is intact.

Obviously, the most significant finding of the physical examination is the change in blood pressure upon standing. This procedure is a test of orthostatic hypotension and provides objective evidence supporting the patient's history and the initial hypothesis. When testing orthostatic changes, it is important to ask the patient about the feeling of lightheadedness to correlate subjective and objective data. There is some controversy about how much of a change in blood pressure or heart rate is diagnostic of orthostatic hypotension, but any change that is coupled with subjective symptoms warrants further evaluation. A drop in systolic blood pressure of more than 20 mm Hg and an increase in pulse rate of greater than 30 beats/min are generally accepted as indications of an orthostatic problem. In this particular case, the heart rate increased significantly (34 beats/min), indicating that the ability of the heart to increase cardiac output via a change in rate is not impaired. This patient may have other problems with her heart that do not allow it to compensate for changes in position; however, the absence of other signs or symptoms of heart failure make this possibility less likely.

The most credible explanation in this case is that her orthostatic hypotension is the result of the antihypertensive medication. Given that the heart is functioning properly, the orthostatic changes would have to be the result of either hypovolemia or impaired vascular constriction. This patient has no history of blood loss or dehydration, which can cause hypovolemia. However, prazosin lowers blood pressure because it impairs peripheral vasoconstriction by blocking α_1-receptors in the vascular smooth muscle.

Virtually all of the antihypertensive medications are capable of causing orthostatic hypotension initially by decreasing blood volume (e.g., diuretics), interfering with vascular constriction (e.g., calcium channel blockers, sympatholytics), or by altering cardiac responsiveness (e.g., sympatholytics); patients should be warned of this potential side effect. This symptom is usually transient and resolves within a few days or weeks. However, in some patients who have had chronically uncontrolled hypertension, this may be a more serious problem. The exact pathology is unclear, but it is likely related to pathologic changes in the walls of blood vessels, such as thickening and stiffening of the vascular medial wall. Whatever the cause, a number of parameters of cardiovascular regulation tend to become "reset" to a higher level in patients who have chronic high blood pressure. The peripheral vasculature is unable to constrict as efficiently over the normal range of blood pressure. In patients such as this, blood pressure can be very difficult to control, and because of medication side effects, compliance may be low. It should be noted that medications are only one cause of impaired vasoconstriction. Alcoholic or diabetic neuropathy, for example, can also lead to orthostatic hypotension.

ASSESSMENT

This patient has **chronic hypertension with symptomatic orthostatic changes** while on the sympatholytic agent prazosin. It would be worth a trial of another antihypertensive medication to see if orthostatic hypotension would subside. At this point, a chart review is warranted to determine which antihypertensive medications she has tried in the past and how effective they were. Her treatment plan involves changing her antihypertensive medication after the blood pressure treatment history has been obtained.

CASE 7-4

INITIAL PRESENTATION
The patient in Case 7-3 presents with the same symptoms.

PHYSICAL EXAMINATION
Her orthostatic vitals are: supine blood pressure, 148/96 mm Hg; and pulse, 82 beats/min; standing blood pressure, 112/74 mm Hg; and pulse, 86 beats/min, with a subjective feeling of lightheadedness after 20 seconds.

12. How do these vital signs change your thinking about possible pathophysiologic mechanisms leading to this person's symptoms?

Discussion
In this case, the heart rate increased after standing up by only 4 beats/min. In a person without cardiovascular problems, an increase in heart rate as small as this would not be a concern. Normally, the increase in peripheral vascular resistance is enough to keep the brain adequately perfused with only minor increases in heart rate. However, the dramatic decrease in blood pressure after standing up and the subjective symptoms in this patient clearly indicate that the brain is not being well perfused. In this patient, the heart should have increased more than 4 beats/min but did not, which indicates a problem with the ability to increase heart rate. A variety of factors, such as the use of β-blockers, cardiomyopathy, and autonomic neuropathy, can interfere with an appropriate increase in heart rate.

ASSESSMENT
This patient has **orthostatic hypotension without an appropriate increase in heart rate**. If she is taking a β-blocker, her medication should be changed. If medication is not the problem, she should be referred to a cardiologist for definitive evaluation.

SUMMARY

Complaints of dizzy spells are common and may be quite puzzling. The etiology is usually benign and self-limiting but also may be serious. The approach to the symptom of dizziness begins with a careful history and then a review of basic physiology. Is the patient having a primary balance problem or a significant decrease in blood perfusion of the brain? If the patient states that rolling over in bed causes a "spinning" sensation, there is certainly a problem with the inner ear. The patient has done nothing to effect an orthostatic change. If, on the other hand, the patient feels like passing out, and the room starts to go dark after sitting up or standing, then there is probably a blood volume problem or at least a relative volume deficit relating to an inability to shunt blood up to the brain when necessary. But determining the cause is not always so easy. Sometimes a perfusion problem may affect the inner ear or the CNS and result in a balance abnormality. Sometimes, despite intensive questioning, the patient cannot decide whether the symptom is best described as imbalance or lightheadedness. Of course, the patient can undergo tests to try to recreate the symptoms and better delineate the problem. Many ear, nose, and throat specialists have tilt chairs with which to perform such testing.

As with all approaches to clinical dilemmas, it is important to establish a priority for all the possibilities. If it seems clear that the patient has BPV, there is time to treat the symptoms and to see if the problem resolves, warning the person of the dangers of falling and advising methods to avoid injury. If it seems likely that the patient has a perfusion deficit related to palpitations or some evidence of emboli, confirming the diagnosis and initiating treatment must be done quickly.

CHAPTER 8
Chief Complaint: Palpitations

CASE 8-1

INITIAL PRESENTATION

Mrs. S., a 36-year-old woman, presents with a chief complaint of "chest palpitations." Mrs. S. reports that her palpitations began 2–3 weeks ago. The episodes occur several times a day and last from a few minutes to roughly an hour. The palpitations are not accompanied by chest pain, nausea, diaphoresis, lightheadedness, or shortness of breath. During the same time period, Mrs. S. has noticed increasing anxiety, and she says this is unusual for her. She has been worried about the welfare of her husband and son, although she admits to having no logical reason for feeling this way. She reports that her job as an office manager has become increasingly more stressful over the past few weeks, and she thinks this possibly could have something to do with her symptoms. Mrs. S. also notes difficulty sleeping recently but states that she is not particularly tired during the day. She has noticed that over the past 2 weeks she is not able to ride her bike as far as she used to because her "legs just get too weak." Mrs. S. suffers from no chronic medical conditions. She takes no medications and does not drink caffeine regularly. Upon further questioning, Mrs. S. admits to having had a severe sore throat roughly 2 months ago. A throat culture at the time was negative, and the sore throat lasted less than 1 week. Two weeks following the sore throat, however, she suffered from severe left-sided neck pain that resolved spontaneously after a few days.

1. What does the term "palpitations" mean?
2. Does the history suggest that anxiety may be causing the palpitations?
3. Could the sore throat and neck pain be related to the current problem?

Discussion

The word "palpitation" is similar to other terms used by lay people such as "dizzy" and "tired," all of which require further definition. Patients often use the word "palpitations" to describe a fast heartbeat, an abnormally strong heartbeat, an irregular heart-

beat, or virtually any condition resulting in the sensation or awareness of one's own heartbeat. Therefore, a patient suffering from
palpitations can have a variety of underlying problems, ranging
from benign to very serious.

Ascertaining the presence or absence of associated cardiac symptoms is important because the relationship can help with the diagnosis and also can indicate the severity of the underlying condition.
The presence of anxiety in this case is likely related to this woman's
"palpitations" because she has no previous history of anxiety. However, without any objective data, it is difficult at this point to
determine any causal relationship between anxiety and palpitations. The patient easily could be increasingly anxious about her
perceived heart problem. On the other hand, the symptom of heart
palpitations is a relatively common physical manifestation of anxiety. Yet another possibility is that both palpitations and anxiety are
related to another factor. Insomnia is similar and could easily be
related to anxiety. However, the sore throat and neck pain may
provide some clues to the pathology of this patient's disorder. It is
certainly possible that the occurrence of these symptoms is coinci-
dental, but a causal relationship should be considered. The temporal association of the two events suggests the first might have
"triggered" the second. This, coupled with the relatively sudden
onset and rapid progression of Mrs. S.'s subsequent symptoms,
makes one think of an infectious or autoimmune pathology.

PHYSICAL EXAMINATION

During the physical examination, the patient's vital signs are:
temperature, 98.9°F; blood pressure, 138/88 mm Hg; pulse, 94
beats/min and regular; and respirations, 16 breaths/min. Mrs. S. is
a thin, somewhat anxious-appearing woman. Her skin is warm and
moist. Her head, eyes, ears, nose, and throat (HEENT) examination
is normal. A small, firm thyroid gland is noted, and her lymph
nodes are normal. There are no carotid bruits. Her lungs are clear to
percussion and auscultation. During her cardiac examination,
there are first (S_1) and second (S_2) heart sounds; no murmurs,
gallops, or rubs are noted. Her abdomen is soft and nontender.
There are no masses or abdominal bruits. Her extremities show no
clubbing, cyanosis, or edema; however, a slight, fine tremor is noted
in both upper extremities. Deep tendon reflexes are all 2+ and
exhibit a rapid return. The remainder of the physical examination is
within normal limits.

4. Do any of the subtle physical findings suggest a pathology?
5. What laboratory tests should be ordered for this patient?

Discussion

It is noteworthy that the patient's pulse is regular. This helps exclude the possibility that the patient suffers from a continuous arrhythmia. The normal cardiac examination is also important because it helps rule out any primary cardiac pathology. The most significant positive findings are the warm, moist skin; tremor; and quick return of deep tendon reflexes, because all of these may signify a thyroid disorder. Thyroid function tests are definitely indicated.

LABORATORY TESTS

An in-office electrocardiogram (ECG) is ordered for Mrs. S., which reveals slight sinus tachycardia in an otherwise normal tracing.

6. What is the significance of the rhythm strip?

Discussion

The ECG strip shows a sinus tachycardia, which may or may not be related to this patient's current medical problem. Rhythm strips are routinely performed in the office when patients complain of palpitations. However, it is important to remember that unless a patient's complaint is continuous, rhythm strips may be normal during intervals between palpitations. In a patient such as this, in whom palpitations occur intermittently, ECG strips may show abnormalities only during an episode. If a cause of the palpitations cannot be determined, patients such as Mrs. S. may need to wear a 24-hour Holter monitor, which continually records a patient's cardiac rhythm.

7. What should be done now in the management of Mrs. S.?

As discussed earlier, a Holter monitor may be used to record a continuous 24-hour tracing of this patient's cardiac rhythm. However, in this particular case, both the history and physical examination have provided some clues as to the cause of Mrs. S.'s problems. The history of difficulty sleeping, anxiety, and muscle weakness are all consistent with hyperthyroidism, a diagnosis that is strongly supported by the objective findings of tachycardia; warm, moist skin; extremity tremor; and rapid return of deep tendon reflexes. Hyperthyroidism caused by either thyroiditis or Graves' disease is much more common in a 36-year-old woman than is heart disease.

The sore throat and subsequent neck pain are common antecedents to thyroiditis. Therefore, it would be reasonable at this point to do some basic thyroid function tests before pursuing other causes of this patient's palpitations. These tests include measuring the levels of triiodothyronine (T_3), thyroxine (T_4), and thyroid-stimulating hormone (TSH). If there were any evidence of a serious arrhythmia, such as a history of syncope, then the Holter monitor should be used immediately. However, in this case, the thyroid tests are less expensive and more likely to solve the problem based on the current information.

The results of the laboratory tests that Mrs. S. underwent are given below. To define her condition further, a radioactive iodine uptake (RAIU) study is also performed. The laboratory tests indicate a hyperthyroid state. This may be caused by true hyperthyroidism (as in Graves' disease or toxic nodular goiter) or to thyroiditis, which is characterized by phases of overactivity (initially) as well as underactivity several weeks after the onset. The history of a sore throat and sore neck as well as her age and sex make subacute thyroiditis a likely possibility.

Laboratory Tests	Patient	Normal Values
T_3	212 ng/dL	70–190 ng/dL
T_4	16.5 µg/dL	5–12 µg/dL
TSH	0.3 mIU/L	0.5–6 mIU/L
RAIU	1% in 24 hrs	10%–30% in 24 hrs

ASSESSMENT

The result of the RAIU study shows that the thyroid gland is not taking up iodine to manufacture thyroid hormones. This seems paradoxical because the blood levels of thyroid hormones are elevated. In thyrotoxicosis caused by Graves' disease or toxic nodules, the iodine uptake corresponds to the blood levels. In patients with thyroiditis, the inflamed gland may leak large amounts of thyroid hormones into the bloodstream and at the same time not be making hormones. This phenomenon accounts for the apparent paradox in the low RAIU study result and the high blood levels of T_3 and T_4. Later in the course of subacute thyroiditis, the reverse may occur, with low levels of T_3 and T_4 and an elevated RAIU study result.

Mrs. S.'s laboratory values are virtually diagnostic of **thyroiditis.** She should be educated as to the usual course of the disorder, which is caused by a virus and should resolve with no specific treatment. A few patients develop long-term hypothyroidism, so the patient should be warned of those symptoms and told to schedule an appointment should they occur.

CASE 8-2

INITIAL PRESENTATION

Mr. K., a 42-year-old man, complains of palpitations that occur intermittently throughout the day. He describes them as a mild sensation of feeling his heart "beat heavily." There are no associated symptoms such as chest pain, shortness of breath, lightheadedness, or diaphoresis. He notes no other cardiac symptoms. Mr. K. was recently diagnosed with hypertension and placed on an α_1-blocker. He has no other medical problems or complaints. There are no precipitating or alleviating factors, and he has no significant family history of heart disease.

PHYSICAL EXAMINATION

The patient's cardiac examination is normal. The remainder of the physical examination is within normal limits. The patient appears healthy but somewhat anxious about his symptoms. His vital signs are: temperature, 98°F; blood pressure, 127/84 mm Hg (sitting); pulse, 90 beats/min and regular; and respirations, 16 breaths/min. On standing, his blood pressure drops to 115/70 mm Hg, and the pulse increases to 104 beats/min. He complains of feeling his heart pound immediately after standing, and this lasts 1–2 minutes. His lungs are clear, and his pulses are full and equal throughout.

ASSESSMENT

One of the major purposes of this book is to explore means of approaching patients' problems. Physicians can use a "systems" or anatomic approach. Unfortunately, such a method may not prove very useful when dealing with a problem that clearly involves a specific system. In this case, it is clear that the cardiac system is involved, at least in part, because palpitations always involve the heart. This is not to say there is intrinsic heart disease, because a rapid or irregular heart rate or excessively strong contractions are often due to extracardiac factors. Thus, other approaches to this patient's problem may be required.

8. What should be done at this point in the management of Mr. K.?

Discussion

One diagnostic approach might be to look up all of the causes of palpitations and proceed to eliminate each cause one by one. The information is usually readily available in any textbook of medicine. Unfortunately, unless the patient's problem happens to be at the top of the list, this process may become quite long, tedious, and expensive.

Another diagnostic approach that is often helpful and also more efficient is to try to categorize a patient's problem as early as possible. Although there are likely dozens of individual causes for palpitations, there are only a few broad categories. Elimination of even a single category eliminates all of the individual etiologies within it. Thus, numerous diagnoses may be discounted with a single history question, physical examination maneuver, or laboratory test. The main problem with such an approach, however, is that appropriate categories must be selected. Fortunately, there are some "golden rules." Of course, one particularly important category, especially in a case involving the heart, is that of an immediately life-threatening disorder. This patient describes mild palpitations that do not involve symptoms of ischemia and that are unaffected by rest or exercise. Although nothing in medicine is ever certain, these are indications that this patient's problem is likely not immediately life-threatening.

Once the physician is comfortable that the patient is relatively safe for the moment, other categories of disease pathology can be ruled in or out. Often, an initial distinction can be made between primary problems, those intrinsic to the affected organ; and secondary problems, those affecting the organ but which are ultimately the result of a more remote pathology. Mrs. S. in Case 8-1, for example, was suffering from an extrinsic cause of palpitations because her heart was being affected by a secondary (thyroid) dysfunction. Her heart was not the primary cause of the problem. Although primary palpitations may not be distinguishable from secondary palpitations definitively without an ECG, historical information often is helpful. When analyzing historical data, there is another golden rule: Never forget a patient's medications as a possible culprit. A variety of medications, such as digitalis, sympathomimetics, theophylline, acetylcholine antagonists, and vasodilating agents (e.g., α_1-blockers) may cause palpitations. This patient recently began using an α_1-blocker for hypertension. This fact, coupled with his relatively mild symptoms and benign medical history, raise the question of palpitations as a side effect of medication. His orthostatic changes in blood pressure and pulse are quite compatible with a side effect of antihypertensive medications.

This patient has **palpitations secondary to an α_1-blocker.** His treatment plan involves changing his medications to a β-blocker. He should call in 1 or 2 days if he has any symptoms and should return for evaluation in 4 weeks. Physicians commonly reevaluate patients in 7–10 days after an antihypertensive medication change, but this is too soon. At least 4 weeks are necessary for the effects of the drug to stabilize.

CASE 8-3

INITIAL PRESENTATION

An 84-year-old woman, Mrs. W., is brought to the emergency department after suffering from palpitations followed by an episode of syncope. Upon further questioning, it is discovered that the patient has had two other episodes similar to this in the past week. The episodes have been associated with mild angina. Her medical history is significant for two previous myocardial infarctions.

PHYSICAL EXAMINATION

The patient is alert and oriented. She is asymptomatic at the time of examination. Her pulse is 52 beats/min and regular. Her cardiac examination is normal. Pedal edema (1+) is noted.

9. How is this case different from Cases 8-1 and 8-2?

Discussion

There are some major differences in this case that distinguish it from the others; and such differences may prove useful for diagnosis and learning. The patient's advanced age is of note. Although this may or may not be related to the current illness, older age is a major risk factor for heart disease. Another major difference is that this patient has a significant history of heart disease that could predispose her to the current condition. Of particular note is that this patient's palpitations are accompanied by other physical manifestations, specifically syncope and angina. Both of these symptoms are indicative of ischemia. This is obviously a concern because this is a sign that these palpitations are interfering with cardiac output. Arrhythmias can decrease cardiac output because the heart is not contracting properly because a rapid heartbeat does not allow for adequate filling time or because it is a symptom of other cardiac disease. Finally, the slow pulse and edema found on physical examination are objective findings that, when coupled with the subjective history, raise concerns about cardiac dysfunction.

10. What should be done in the management of Mrs. W.?

There is no evidence to suggest that Mrs. W. has a secondary cause of palpitations, as in the previous case. Therefore, an ECG tracing of her cardiac rhythm during an episode would be very helpful. Because of this patient's advanced age and potentially serious problems, an admission for cardiac workup would be safer than sending her home with a Holter monitor. In addition, an ECG tracing while she is symptom free might also be helpful, given her bradycardia.

Several ECGs are performed, and the results are crucial for diagnosis. The testing confirmed that Mrs. W.'s palpitations were related to and most certainly caused by her arrhythmias. In one tracing, her ventricular rate varied from 120–280 beats/min. The QRS complexes were normal, indicating that electrical conduction through the ventricles is occurring in a normal pattern. In other words, the ventricles appear to be unaffected by the disorder. The tachycardia is occurring because rapid impulses are being generated somewhere above the ventricles (i.e., supraventricular tachycardia [SVT]). As discussed previously, any disturbance of cardiac rhythm can result in palpitations, thus explaining one of this woman's subjective complaints. Another tracing shows an irregularly irregular rhythm, the hallmark of atrial fibrillation. After this pattern ends, there is a period of asystole that lasts several seconds before the sinus node recovers. No heartbeat for several seconds would account for her syncope. These two tracings indicate that the problem with the electrical conduction originates in the atria. However, it is a third tracing that is probably the most helpful in making a unifying diagnosis.

In the third strip, there are no P waves, which indicates a lack of atrial depolarization. In fact, there is no activity at all other than depolarization and repolarization of the ventricles. This explains her bradycardia and suggests a diagnosis. Because there is no atrial activity (sinus arrest), it can be concluded that the sinoatrial (SA) node is not functioning correctly. Ventricular activity is the result of an "escape" rhythm generated in the atrioventricular (AV) node. This "back-up" mechanism takes over when the SA node fails to send a signal to the ventricles at least 35–40 times/min. The AV node has an intrinsic rate of approximately 30 beats/min, which is not enough to allow full bodily function but is enough to prevent death. These tracings are diagnostic of the sick sinus syndrome. This disorder is characterized by bradycardia or periods of asystole due to dysfunction of the SA node. Intermittent SVT, atrial fibrillation, or other arrhythmias generated in the SA node are not uncommon with the sick sinus syndrome.

ASSESSMENT

Mrs. W. does have significant heart disease manifested by various rhythm disturbances, and she is diagnosed with **sick sinus syndrome.** The associated rate changes cause the sensation of palpitations. The slow rates as well as the very fast rates do not allow adequate blood volume to be pumped to the coronary arteries, and this results in angina. When there is a several-second period of asystole, the brain becomes starved for oxygen, and syncope occurs. Her treatment plan includes admittance to the hospital for close monitoring and a cardiology consultation. She may well require an artificial pacemaker.

CASE 8-4

INITIAL PRESENTATION

Ms. L., a 49-year-old woman, is complaining of intermittent palpitations that began roughly 2 months ago. Her symptoms occur intermittently throughout the day. She reports no dyspnea, chest pain, or loss of consciousness. She notes increasing fatigue during the past 2 months. She has no history of cardiac disease. Mrs. L. states that she has an appointment with her gynecologist for increased menstrual bleeding over the past several months.

PHYSICAL EXAMINATION

During the physical examination, Ms. L. has a normal temperature, a blood pressure of 110/74 mm Hg, and a regular pulse of 104 beats/min. Her mucous membranes appear slightly dry and pale. The remainder of the physical examination is within normal limits.

ASSESSMENT

It may be a bit obvious when presented this way with only the pertinent positives and negatives noted. Unfortunately, real patients rarely give such succinct histories. This case should be looked at in terms of a secondary versus primary cardiac problem. As with some of the other cases, this patient's presentation appears relatively benign and is not associated with other cardiac symptoms. Furthermore, she has no history of heart disease. All of these factors tend to decrease the possibility of a primary cardiac problem. The increased menstrual blood loss, fatigue, and physical examination findings of pale mucosa suggest the possibility of **anemia.** To rule out primary heart disease, an ECG tracing while palpitations are occurring would be necessary. A reasonable first step, however, would be to check Ms. L.'s hematocrit. Anemia results in decreased oxygen-carry capacity of the blood. To deliver the required oxygen to tissues, the heart compensates by increasing its rate. A heart rate that seems to the patient to be abnormally rapid for a given level of activity may be perceived as palpitations.

CASE 8-5

INITIAL PRESENTATION

Ms. D., a 38-year-old woman, complains of palpitations with any form of exercise. She has noted this phenomenon for more than 1 year, and her previous primary care physician told her it was caused by stress. Although her job as a lawyer is indeed stressful, she says that her stress level has not increased during the past year. She is an avid runner but recently has been unable to even walk fast without a very bothersome pounding in her chest and a feeling of weakness. She also notes frequent generalized headaches. Her previous physician suggested the possibility of reactive hypoglycemia, but a low-carbohydrate diet has not helped. Her previous physician had her wear a Holter monitor for 1 day, but it showed only occasional tachycardia appropriate for the degree of exercise at the time. An exercise treadmill test, which she performed while under the care of her previous physician, was negative, except for the fact that her heart rate increased more than expected for the amount of physical stress, and her blood pressure increased more than normal. When her previous physician suggested she take tranquilizers, she lost faith in him. She is now seeking the advice of a new physician.

11. As this patient's new physician, what is the first step in her care?

Discussion

The physician takes a very careful history and finds that emotional stress has also caused palpitations; however, unlike the first 37 years of her life, the palpitations are now disabling and often accompanied by headache and weakness. During a recent court case, the patient became pale and diaphoretic and had to have one of her partners finish her cross-examination. Her partner said that not only her face but also her hands were snow white. The physician finds that she has no history of any illnesses of consequence and takes no medications on a regular basis. She has a family history that is negative for cardio-vascular disease as well as thyroid disorders.

PHYSICAL EXAMINATION

She appears well and healthy with good color. Her vital signs are normal. However, her pulse goes up to 140 beats/min with only 2 minutes of light running in place. Following exercise, her blood pressure is 168/100 mm Hg, and she appears to be rather pale (especially her hands and feet). Her heart sounds are normal. Her reflexes are normal with no evidence of a faster-than-normal return. Her fundi show no evidence of disease. The remainder of her examination is completely normal.

The patient's complete blood count, chemistry screen, and thyroid tests are normal. The ECG and Holter monitor results from her previous physician are reviewed and agreed to be normal.

12. What might cause the elevated blood pressure and pulse along with the blanching of her extremities?

Discussion

A powerful vasoconstrictor can cause the blood pressure to elevate and the skin to blanch. Depending on the type of substance, the heart rate might go up, down, or stay the same. The patient denies taking any medications or drugs, and the physician finds no evidence on examination or laboratory tests that she has hyperthyroidism. The physician then considers endogenous vasoconstrictors, such as catecholamines. If her adrenal medulla were overactive and producing too much epinephrine or norepinephrine, the result might be the signs and symptoms that have been recorded. Stress alone for some people can cause a significant outpouring of catecholamines, and exercise can cause the pulse and blood pressure to rise substantially. However, her symptoms are new over the past year and must be explained on the basis of a change in her life style, an altered reaction to stress, or a physiologic difference. Her husband says she has had no emotional changes recently other than what would be expected in someone who was not able to do the things she did previously without experiencing disabling palpitations.

> 13. What pathology of the adrenal glands might cause an episodic excess in catecholamines?

A tumor of the adrenal medulla called a pheochromocytoma can cause extreme vasoconstriction and dangerous elevations in blood pressure. Headache and blanching of the extremities may also occur, as well as palpitations. The signs and symptoms vary depending on the relative amounts of the two hormones that are produced. The physician measures her 24-hour urinary catecholamine level and finds it to be markedly elevated. He then orders a magnetic resonance imaging scan of the adrenal glands, which reveals a 6-cm mass in the left adrenal gland.

ASSESSMENT

The patient is diagnosed with **pheochromocytoma.** The physician places her on an α-blocker and warns her to avoid physically and emotionally stressful situations until a definitive treatment can be effected. A surgeon who is experienced in pheochromocytoma removal is scheduled to evaluate the patient.

SUMMARY

Palpitations are merely the awareness of one's own heartbeat. Therefore, it is helpful to get as accurate a description as possible of the nature of the cardiac sensation. When approaching such a patient, it is necessary to determine whether the events are primary (originating in the heart) or secondary (the heart is responding with an arrhythmia as a result of another organ system dysfunction). Some secondary causes include the following:

- Medical problems such as anemia, anxiety disorders, dehydration, pheochromocytoma, fever, and thyrotoxicosis
- Medications such as vasodilators, amphetamines, theophylline, beta agonists, phenothiazines, and antiarrhythmics
- Drugs such as caffeine, alcohol, nicotine, and cocaine

Primary causes of palpitations include any electrical or mechanical dysfunction in the heart. When a primary cause is suspected, an ECG tracing is often the most helpful for definitive diagnosis. If the patient is symptom free while being evaluated, a 24-hour Holter monitor may be required to record an event.

CHAPTER 9
Chief Complaint: Cough

CASE 9-1

INITIAL PRESENTATION

Ms. J., a 44-year-old woman, presents as a new patient. She states that she has had a cough for the last several years, which she feels has not changed. The cough is worse in the morning and is productive of a small bit of white sputum. She denies fever or hemoptysis. She does admit to slight shortness of breath on exertion for several years but otherwise admits to no other symptoms.

> Chronic, constant, productive cough

1. What is the basic mechanism of a cough?

Discussion

Cough is a general response to irritation of the bronchial tubes and is the body's attempt to clear the cause of such irritation. A cough is preceded by a prolonged inspiration and complete closure of the glottis. Then, sudden contraction of accessory respiratory muscles causes a sudden opening of the glottis followed by rapid expulsion of air. During a cough, bronchial tubes constrict, reducing their diameter and thus increasing the velocity of the expired air. Virtually anything that can irritate bronchial airways can result in a cough.

2. How does the pattern of this presentation assist with diagnosis in this patient?

Because any bronchial tube irritant can potentially result in cough, the constant and prolonged nature of the patient's symptoms would suggest an indolent, chronic pathology. In addition, the productive nature of the cough tends to support involvement of secretory cells, such as the goblet cells in the respiratory epithelium. Sputum examination often can help significantly with the diagnosis. Greenish or yellow sputum often implies an infectious etiology, whereas brown or red sputum usually indicates the presence of blood. It is reasonable to collect sputum samples from patients to help isolate an organism when an infectious etiology is suspected. However, in this case, the white-colored sputum and prolonged course, along with the absence of other associated symptoms (e.g., fever), make infection less likely. Thus, a sputum sample would most likely be of low yield.

The patient's medical history includes the usual childhood illnesses but no chronic adult illnesses, surgeries, or hospitalizations. She has no allergies.

Ms. J. had menarche at age 12 years, and her periods have been regular since then. She has had a total of seven sexual partners and has always used condoms for birth control. She denies any history of sexually transmitted diseases (STDs). She is not currently sexually active. The patient was married for 10 years but was divorced 15 years ago. She currently lives alone. She has had several relationships since her marriage but nothing "serious." She states that she has many friends and enjoys an active social life. She currently works as a legal secretary. Ms. J. has an occasional glass of wine with dinner and drinks two or three beers when out on a weekend night. She has smoked 2–3 packs of cigarettes a day since she was 18 years old. She has never used illicit drugs. Her two brothers, ages 46 and 47 years, are alive and well. Her father and mother are both in their 60s and have no medical problems of which she is aware. All of her grandparents have died of "natural causes." She is unaware of any significant family diseases.

The patient has no history of asthma or other lung disease of which she is aware. She denies hemoptysis, wheezing, and shortness of breath other than as mentioned in the history of the present illness. She has no known heart problems. She denies orthopnea, paroxysmal nocturnal dyspnea (PND), edema, and chest pain. The remainder of the review of systems is unremarkable.

3. How has the medical history helped with a diagnosis in this patient?
4. Is this information mostly positive or negative?

This patient's medical history is largely unremarkable and helps exclude cardiac or infectious etiologies. Her smoking habit is probably the most notable aspect of her history, and it is particularly important as a risk factor for pulmonary problems. In the lung, smoking increases the risk for cancer, bronchitis, pneumonia, and emphysema.

PHYSICAL EXAMINATION

This is a well-developed, well-nourished woman who appears generally healthy. Her vital signs are: pulse, 76 beats/min; blood pressure, 110/70 mm Hg; temperature, 98°F; and respirations, 18 breaths/min. Her skin, hair, and nails are normal. Head, ears, eyes, nose, and throat (HEENT) examination is normal. The thyroid is normal, and there is no cervical lymphadenopathy. Heart examination reveals no murmurs, rubs, or gallops. Her lungs are clear except for a slight increase in her bronchial sounds. Her abdominal examination is unremarkable. Her extremities are normal, without clubbing or cyanosis. The neurologic system is normal.

LABORATORY RESULTS

A chest radiograph is normal. No infiltrates or masses are present. A bronchodilator did not result in any significant change. Results of the pulmonary function tests (PFTs) are given below.

Pulmonary Function Test	Predicted	Actual	% Predicted
Forced vital capacity (FVC)	2.39	2.08	87
Forced expiratory volume at one second (FEV_1)	1.98	1.08	55
FEV_1/FVC	83	52	. . .

5. Are these results specific and abnormal enough to help focus the diagnostic pathway?
6. What would be the expected value for the residual volume (RV) in this patient?

Discussion

The normal chest radiograph helps rule out chronic disorders such as congestive heart failure (CHF) or neoplasm as the potential causes of this woman's cough, but otherwise it is not terribly helpful. The PFTs, however, are extremely valuable. Although both the FVC and the FEV_1 are decreased, the FEV_1 is disproportionately small, indicating an obstructive disorder.

The RV is the volume of air that remains in the lungs after a maximal forced expiration. The ratio of FEV_1/FVC indicates an obstructive disorder, which means that some pathologic process is obstructing the expiration of air. In other words, air is being trapped in the lungs. Thus, one would expect the RV to be increased in this patient.

ASSESSMENT

7. What is the diagnosis at this point?
8. What factors led to this conclusion?

Discussion

There are three major subsets of chronic obstructive pulmonary disease (COPD): asthma, emphysema, and chronic bronchitis. Variant forms of asthma can certainly present as a cough. However, asthma is caused by an allergic response in which bronchial tubes are constricted. Thus, asthma would be suspected if the PFTs had improved after bronchodilation, but this did not occur. Emphysema is a pathology in which alveolar walls are destroyed with enlargement of air spaces distal to the terminal bronchioles. Smoking does increase this woman's chances of developing emphysema, especially if she had a predisposing factor, such as a positive family history. In addition, asthma, emphysema, and chronic bronchitis often overlap. In this case, however, the clinical picture is really one of predominant bronchitis. In fact, the clinical definition of chronic bronchitis is the presence of a productive cough on most days for at least 3 months of the year for a minimum of 2 years in succession. Chronic bronchitis increases in prevalence with the cumulative number of cigarettes an individual smokes. It is very common for heavy smokers to have a productive cough, which may or may not signify bronchitis. In this case, however, the history of slight dyspnea and the PFT results clearly indicate some degree of bronchial narrowing.

9. How should this patient be treated?

Other than supplemental oxygen therapy for people who are hypoxic and attention to other risk factors, there is very little that can be done to treat chronic bronchitis other than help this patient to **stop smoking.** Smoking cessation often results in decreased symptom severity with occasional complete resolution. In addition, smoking cessation should decrease the likelihood of progressive damage to her lung tissue. Patients with chronic bronchitis do not clear pulmonary secretions as well as those with normal bronchi and, thus, they are prone to pneumonia. Ms. J. suffers from **chronic bronchitis.** Her treatment plan involves a smoking cessation program and a pneumococcal vaccine injection.

CASE 9-2

INITIAL PRESENTATION

Mr. T., a 34-year-old man, complains of a chronic nonproductive cough. His cough has persisted intermittently for several years. He reports no associated shortness of breath, chest pain, or fever. He has suffered from "heartburn" for many years, which is usually relieved with an antacid. He drinks 3–6 beers a day and has a 10-pack-year history of smoking. Previous hospitalizations include a bout of pneumonia last year.

PHYSICAL EXAMINATION

During his physical examination, the patient coughs intermittently, and the stool guaiac test is positive. His physical examination is otherwise unremarkable.

10. How might Mr. T.'s heartburn and cough be related?

Discussion

As in the case of Ms. J., this man's cough is chronic, suggesting an indolent process affecting the lungs. Virtually anything capable of irritating bronchial tissues can result in cough. Associated symptoms, then, can be very useful in coming to a diagnosis. This patient complains of "heartburn." In addition, he has a significant history of alcohol intake and smoking, both of which are risk factors for gastroesophageal reflux disease (GERD). This disorder is extremely common, even in individuals without such risk factors. Fortunately, most cases respond favorably to intermittent treatment with antacids. However, roughly 1 in 10 patients fails to get relief with antacids and requires further treatment with type 2 histamine (H_2) blockers, sucralfate, or, in severe cases, proton-pump inhibitors with omeprazole. In these cases, definitive diagnosis may require endoscopy and biopsy. Patients with GERD also should be educated about foods and habits that increase gastric acid secretion or decrease low esophageal sphincter pressure, such as alcohol, smoking, and fatty foods. Although the disorder is usually benign in its course, it should be controlled as well as possible. Occasionally, aspiration of gastric reflux during sleep results in chronic bronchial irritation and cough, as is likely in this patient. Recent studies suggest that cough is fairly common in people with prolonged GERD. There also is evidence that prolonged exposure of the esophageal lining to gastric contents increases the risk of Barrett's esophagitis and adenocarcinoma of the esophagus. A small number of patients with severe, persistent esophagitis may require surgical intervention.

ASSESSMENT

Mr. T. has a **chronic cough secondary to GERD.** His treatment plan includes antireflux measures as discussed above. Elevation of the head of the bed also may be very helpful. Mr. T. should also be advised to quit smoking and limit his alcohol intake to one drink a day.

CASE 9-3

INITIAL PRESENTATION

Ms. J. (Case 9-1) returns 8 years later at age 52 years complaining of a worsening of her cough. She stopped smoking 4 years ago after another exacerbation of chronic bronchitis. Her cough steadily decreased over the past several years but never quite resolved. She now notes that the cough has been increasing in severity again over the past month. The cough is not productive of mucus. She has no chills or fever, and she reports no shortness of breath, wheezing, or orthopnea.

PHYSICAL EXAMINATION

Ms. J.'s weight, compared to that of 3 months ago, reveals a 5-lb loss. The remainder of the physical examination is unremarkable.

LABORATORY TESTS

Laboratory results indicate that her complete blood count (CBC) is within normal limits. A chest radiograph shows a 2–4-cm area of consolidation in her left upper lobe near the hilum. There is no evidence of pleural effusion or other infiltrates.

ASSESSMENT

11. What is the leading diagnosis now?

Discussion

Ms. J.'s history of smoking puts her at risk for a variety of pulmonary disorders. Cessation of smoking usually retards the progression of chronic bronchitis or other forms of COPD but not always. In addition, Ms. J. is also at risk for pulmonary infection such as pneumonia. However, the absence of other respiratory symptoms and the normal white blood cell (WBC) count makes this condition less likely. It is also worth noting that her cough is not productive at this point. A change in a chronic cough, particularly in a patient with a smoking history, should raise the concern of pulmonary neoplasia. A biopsy is required to confirm this diagnosis, but a solid mass on the chest radiograph supports such a diagnosis. Weight loss also is consistent with a chronic disorder such as lung cancer. Pulmonary neoplasms can present in a variety of ways, including symptoms of chest pain, dyspnea, weight loss, and cough. This is an example of a situation in which cough is produced by a simple mechanical irritation of bronchial epithelium. Occasionally, bronchogenic carcinoma is associated with paraneoplastic syndromes. Increased levels of antidiuretic hormone (ADH), adrenocorticotropic hormone (ACTH), parathyroid hormone (PTH), prostaglandins, gonadotropins, calcitonin, or serotonin can cause laboratory abnormalities even before symptoms are noted. Unfortunately, pulmonary carcinomas are usually rapidly progressive. Although localized, small, solitary tumors can be cured with surgical intervention, many patients have distant metastases upon detection, which makes cure much less likely. In this case, immediate surgical and oncologic consults are warranted to assess prognosis and begin treatment.

A **lung mass** is seen on radiograph of a patient with a chronic cough and a smoking history. **Squamous cell carcinoma** is most likely. The treatment plan consists of referral to a thoracic surgeon.

CASE 9-4

INITIAL PRESENTATION

A 44-year-old Mexican man complains of a progressively worsening cough over the past 5 months. His cough is associated with shortness of breath on exertion over the past year. He must sleep propped up on two to three pillows to breathe (i.e., he has two- to three-pillow orthopnea). He notes PND intermittently. The patient has lived in a very rural area of Mexico for most of his life. His medical history is significant for several episodes of sore throat as a child.

PHYSICAL EXAMINATION

Examination of the lungs reveals bilateral basilar crackles but is otherwise clear to percussion and auscultation. A cardiac examination reveals a prominent first heart sound (S_1). A soft (I/VI) holosystolic murmur is heard at the apex. The second heart sound (S_2) is normal. There is a loud opening snap. A soft diastolic murmur is heard best at the apex and left axilla. There is no jugular venous distention and no peripheral edema. The remainder of the physical examination is within normal limits. An electrocardiogram (ECG) shows notched P waves, but is otherwise normal. A chest radiograph shows bilateral costodiaphragmatic angle blunting. The left atrium appears slightly enlarged. The lung fields are otherwise clear.

12. What pathophysiologic conditions are suggested by the abnormal physical examination and laboratory findings?
13. What cardiac disease might result in these pathophysiologic changes?

Discussion

This appears to be a chronic, progressive problem. Although a variety of primary lung pathologies could present with a similar timing pattern, the associated symptoms of PND and orthopnea are indicative of left-sided heart failure. The bilateral basilar crackles suggest the presence of interstitial lung fluid, and blunting of the costophrenic angles on chest radiograph indicates some pleural effusion. The bilateral findings are important because they eliminate a localized etiology. Pneumonia, for example, may result in pleural effusion, but it is usually confined to the side of the pulmonary infection. However, this is not a "typical" presentation for CHF. Most commonly, CHF presents in older individuals with known heart disease or hypertension. In addition, the absence of peripheral edema and jugular venous distention suggests that the right heart is not yet affected. This case is a good example of the importance of considering epidemiologic risk factors and physical examination findings. The loud S_1 and the opening snap both indicate a pathology involving the mitral or tricuspid valves. This also is supported by the diastolic murmur, suggesting stenosis of one or both of these valves. Radiation of these sounds to the apex and axilla help localize the problem to the mitral valve. The holosystolic murmur also implies some degree of mitral regurgitation as well. Notched P waves on the ECG and left atrial enlargement on chest radiograph are consistent with atrial hypertrophy, which could result from chronic increased atrial pressure as the result of atrial muscle pushing against a stenotic mitral valve.

ASSESSMENT

14. Assuming this man has mitral valve disease, what might have caused it?
15. How could his disease have caused his cough?

Discussion

A potentially important aspect of this man's history is that he is Mexican and has lived most of his life in a rural community. Areas such as this may be relatively underserved by the medical community. As a result, this man may not have received the same medical care as other patients. The sparse history of recurrent sore throats might suggest multiple streptococcal infections. Normally, penicillin is given to patients with "strep throat" to prevent poststreptococcal glomerulonephritis and rheumatic heart disease. If this individual did not receive prophylactic antibiotic treatment, rheumatic heart disease is certainly a possibility. In this case, as in any case of left-sided heart failure, cough is caused by irritation of bronchial tissues due to the accumulation of fluid that is not being appropriately cleared from the lungs by the left heart. In this patient, echocardiography is recommended to determine the extent of valve dysfunction prior to surgical replacement. It also should be noted that patients with atrial hypertrophy and distention are also at risk for atrial fibrillation.

This man is diagnosed with **rheumatic heart disease** with mitral stenosis. His treatment plan includes an echocardiogram and a cardiac surgery consult.

CASE 9-5

INITIAL PRESENTATION

A 66-year-old woman complains of coughing up blood. A cough began insidiously 2 months ago, but she began coughing up bright red blood yesterday. She also notes anorexia with a 5–10-lb weight loss over the past 6 months. Night sweats have been present intermittently over the same period of time. She has no other significant medical history.

PHYSICAL EXAMINATION

The woman appears chronically ill. She has a temperature of 100.2°F. A lung examination reveals slight dullness to percussion and crackles in the right upper lobe. Otherwise, her lungs are clear to percussion and auscultation. Her heart is beating at a regular rate. No murmurs, gallops, or rubs are detected. The remainder of the physical examination is within normal limits.

LABORATORY TESTS

A chest radiograph shows a right posterior apical infiltrate. A CBC indicates her WBC count is 12,000 cells/mm³ with increased neutrophils (normal, 4500–11,000 cells/mm³).

16. What kinds of pathologic processes could cause her symptoms and signs?

Discussion

Hemoptysis occurs when damage to the pulmonary parenchyma becomes severe enough to cause bleeding into the alveolar or bronchial spaces. Increased temperature and a high neutrophil count strongly suggest a bacterial infection, making some type of pneumonia likely in this case. It is quite possible that this woman is suffering from a common bacterial pneumonia such as that caused by *Streptococcus pneumoniae*. However, there are a number of aspects of this patient's history that raise concerns of more indolent infections such as a fungus or tuberculosis (TB). Although virtually any type of bacterial pneumonia can cause hemoptysis if severe enough, this is a very common finding in patients with TB. In addition, most common bacterial pneumonias progress rapidly within hours to days. This patient's cough began 2 months ago, and her night sweats and weight loss have been present for 6 months. Weight loss is a common characteristic of virtually any chronic illness. Night sweats are similarly indicative of a wide variety of illnesses, although this is a common symptom of TB. The chest radiograph also may help support a diagnosis of TB because involvement of the apical regions is most common. Unfortunately, definitive diagnosis can be difficult. Tuberculin skin tests are positive in most immunocompetent patients with reactivated disease. However, reactivated TB is much more prevalent in immunocompromised individuals who may be anergic, thus dramatically increasing the rate of false-negative results. In patients with a strong pretest probability, the presence of acid-fast bacilli in sputum virtually confirms the diagnosis. However, sputum samples also should be cultured in all cases because of the possibility of nontuberculin mycobacterial infections, the relatively low sensitivity of sputum stain, and the need to assess the sensitivity of the organism to pharmacologic agents.

17. Assuming this patient has TB, when was she most likely infected?

Tuberculosis still is a major health problem around the world. It is more common in Third World countries, but after a low several years ago, it is becoming increasingly more common and harder to treat in the United States. The HIV epidemic also has resulted in increasing cases of *Mycobacterium avium-intracellulare*. TB is interesting and somewhat puzzling because of its extremely variable clinical course. Most patients are completely asymptomatic upon initial infection, as this patient probably was. Occasionally, however, initial infection causes cough, fever, lung infiltration, or pleural effusion. Most individuals are infected at a relatively young age. Roughly 5%–10% of the United States population has positive skin tests but are asymptomatic. After primary infection, the organism is usually "walled off" by the immune system, and most of the organisms are killed. In some patients, however, reactivation of the disease occurs with older age or if the person becomes immunocompromised. Reactivated TB is the most common form of clinical disease. The disease can present almost anywhere in the body, but it is most common in the lungs.

ASSESSMENT

18. How should this patient be treated if a definitive diagnosis of TB is obtained?

Discussion

TB is growing increasingly less sensitive to chemotherapy and therefore increasingly more difficult to treat. A major part of therapy includes prevention of disease spread. Treatment of pulmonary TB requires immediate hospitalization and isolation because of the high risk of contagion. In addition, the Centers for Disease Control and Prevention must be informed, and anyone in close contact with the patient should be given tuberculin skin tests repeatedly. First-line antibiotic therapy consists of isoniazid, rifampin, and pyrazinamide. Second-line therapy consists of ethambutol and streptomycin. In patients with active TB, multiple antibiotic therapy is necessary because of increasing resistance of the organism to these agents.

Fungal infections of the lung can be clinically indistinguishable from pulmonary TB. Histoplasmosis, coccidioidomycosis, and others have less predilection for the upper lobes than does TB; however, in an individual case, this and other differences are not helpful. Skin tests and sputum cultures for fungus and TB are essential.

This woman had acid-fast bacilli in her sputum, and cultures were positive for *Mycobacterium tuberculosis*. The positive sputum stain is virtually confirmative of **tuberculosis** in a patient with this clinical picture. She will be started on triple antibiotic therapy and hospitalized at a facility with experience in treating TB.

SUMMARY

Cough is a defense function that can help rid the lungs of irritants. Any noxious external substance as well as many internal products, such as stomach secretions or blood, may serve as an irritant. Excessive amounts of normal bronchial secretions caused by the reaction to infections or allergies also can trigger the cough reflex.

As with other pathologic conditions, a logical analysis of the historical, physical, and laboratory findings helps focus the diagnostic process. Determining whether the disorder is chronic or acute, indolent or virulent, isolated to the lung or associated with other organ system abnormalities are all important in making a rapid, cost-effective diagnosis so that treatment may be initiated.

CHAPTER 10
Chief Complaint: Diarrhea and Constipation

CASE 10-1

INITIAL PRESENTATION

Mrs. S., a 30-year-old Jewish housewife, presents with a chief complaint of persistent diarrhea. The patient reports that she has had intermittent diarrhea for more than 2 months. She reports three to five loose or watery stools a day accompanied by mild abdominal cramping. She also occasionally notices blood and mucus in her stools. She frequently experiences an urgency to defecate. The symptoms tend to wax and wane over several weeks and are not associated with any specific dietary intake, including dairy products or sugars. During more severe episodes, she occasionally notices mild fever. She has no history of travel outside of the country or of exposure to uncooked food or contaminated water of any kind. Mrs. S. states that before the onset of her diarrhea, she had suffered from constipation for several years. During this period, she also noticed some mucus and blood in her stools. She only recently became worried when she read in a magazine that diarrhea and blood in the stool are potential signs of colon cancer. Her husband reports that Mrs. S. has been noticeably more tired in the last year. She has never smoked or used drugs. She currently takes no medications and drinks alcohol only occasionally. She has had a monogamous relationship with her husband for the past 12 years. She denies any significant psychiatric instability and does not consider herself to be an overly anxious person. Her husband supports this assessment. The patient denies heat intolerance, tremor, muscular weakness, significant weight loss, and any other symptoms of hyperthyroidism. Mrs. S. has had no hospitalizations or surgeries. She states that she has never been worried about her weight and has never tried extensive dieting measures. The patient has no family history of colon cancer, but she does have an aunt who also has chronic diarrhea.

> **Chronic diarrhea**

> **Absence of risk factors and the chronic nature of the symptoms make infection less likely.**

1. What is diarrhea, and how should questioning of the patient proceed?

Discussion

Clinically, diarrhea is defined as an increase in the frequency,
volume, or water content of a patient's stools. A precise definition
of a patient's complaint is always helpful. The pathogenesis of
diarrhea is varied, but generally can be attributed to an increase of
secretions into the gastrointestinal (GI) tract, a decrease in the
absorption from the GI tract, or an increase in GI motility. Diag-
nostically, however, it may be more helpful to categorize diarrhea as
chronic or acute, and infectious or noninfectious. Diarrhea is a
common patient complaint, and initial differentiation between the
various types of diarrhea can be a very effective diagnostic aid.

2. Does the history suggest an infectious etiology?
3. Is a malignancy likely?

This patient is complaining of chronic diarrhea (lasting more
than 3 weeks), which helps eliminate but does not totally preclude
an infectious etiology. Most infectious cases of diarrhea are rather
acute. Exceptions to this are *Giardia lamblia, Clostridia difficile*, and
the various diseases associated with HIV infection. This patient
does not have any obvious risk factors for a chronic infectious
disease. The patient's history also is significant for a number of
pertinent negative factors that are discussed later in this chapter. Of
"positive" significance, however, is the presence of blood in the
stool, which clearly implies direct damage to the tissues of the GI
tract. Chronic bloody diarrhea usually suggests immunosuppression, medication use (particularly antibiotics), colon cancer or
polyps, radiation exposure, or inflammatory bowel disease. This
case illustrates again the importance of a careful risk factor assessment. Although she is worried about colon cancer and the possibility cannot be overlooked given the consequences, neoplasms of
the colon are very rare in a woman her age unless she has one of the
rare familial polyposis conditions of the colon. In addition, she has
no known history of immunosuppression, medication use, or radiation exposure. At this point, therefore, inflammatory bowel disease is a leading hypothesis.

PHYSICAL EXAMINATION

The patient's vital signs are: blood pressure, 130/74 mm Hg; pulse,
76 beats/min; respirations, 16 breaths/min; temperature, 99°F. The

patient is a well-developed woman in no apparent distress. A head, ears, eyes, nose, and throat (HEENT) examination is unremarkable. Her mucous membranes are moist and without pallor. Her neck is supple and shows no thyromegaly. The patient's chest and lungs are clear to auscultation. Her heart rate is regular without murmurs, gallops, or rubs. Her abdomen is soft with no organomegaly. There is a slight tenderness to deep palpation in the lower quadrants. Her extremities show no clubbing, cyanosis, or edema. Her skin has a normal texture and no rashes. A rectal examination reveals normal sphincter tone. No hemorrhoids are noted; the stool is guaiac positive. A neurologic examination is unremarkable.

4. How has the physical examination helped in forming a diagnosis?

Discussion

As is often the case in internal medicine, the physical examination has confirmed many of the positive and negative aspects of the history. The normal pulse rate and absence of dryness or pallor of the mucous membranes give some indication that blood loss has not been great, because these factors suggest that she is not anemic. The normal skin and thyroid size help rule out hyperthyroidism as a potential cause. Mild tenderness in the lower abdominal quadrants is consistent with a nonspecific inflammatory process in the lower GI tract. The positive guaiac is not surprising given this patient's history, and the absence of hemorrhoids helps rule this out as a potential source of the bleeding.

LABORATORY TESTS

A number of laboratory tests were ordered. The results are given below.

Laboratory Tests	Patient	Normal Values
Complete blood cell count (CBC) with differential		
White blood cells (WBCs)	10,200 cells/mm^3	4800–10,800 cells/mm^3
Segmented neutrophils	76%	31%–71%
Bands	14%	0–12%
Lymphocytes	7%	15%–48%
Monocytes	2%	3%–10%
Eosinophils	1%	0–7%
Basophils	0	0–2%
Hemoglobin	11 g/dL	12–16 g/dL
Hematocrit	34%	35%–45%
Mean corpuscular volume (MCV)	78 fL	80–100 fL
Erythrocyte sedimentation rate (ESR)	55 mm/hr	0–20 mm/hr

A stool sample shows some gross blood and numerous neutrophils on microscopic examination. Examination of stool for ova,
parasites, and bacteria reveals no pathogens.

**5. Does the laboratory work suggest inflammation? If so, is
there a diagnosis? If not, what is the next step?**

Discussion

The CBC shows a slight leukocytosis with a very slight microcytic
anemia. These findings are consistent with an inflammatory process and chronic blood loss. The absence of ova, parasites, and
bacterial pathogens helps rule out an infectious etiology. The presence of neutrophils in the stool sample again suggests an inflammatory process involving the GI tract. Unfortunately, this test has a
relatively low specificity. The erythrocyte sedimentation rate (ESR)
is the rate at which red blood cells (RBCs) settle out of unclotted
blood. It is an indicator of an inflammatory process. Inflammatory
mediators cause RBCs to aggregate and fall out of suspension more
quickly. The problem with the ESR is that it is nonspecific. Virtually
any systemic inflammatory process can increase the ESR.

All of the laboratory reports suggest a diagnosis of inflammatory
bowel disease as the cause of Mrs. S.'s diarrhea. However, direct
visualization of the colon is crucial for a definitive diagnosis whenever the cause of bleeding has not been identified. Although cancer
is unlikely, missing it would be devastating. In addition, the cause
of the inflammatory process has yet to be determined. A sigmoidoscopy with mucosal biopsy is necessary at this point.

A sigmoidoscopy reveals a friable mucosa with generalized co-
lonic involvement consisting of 1-mm lesions that bleed after swab-
bing with cotton. Biopsy shows small, superficial ulcerations that
do not extend into the submucosa. There is no evidence of ischemia. A cotton swab specimen shows no evidence of amebae or other
parasites, and a bacterial culture is negative.

6. How should the physician proceed?

In the absence of infection or ischemia, there are two principal
causes of generalized inflammatory bowel disease: ulcerative colitis
and Crohn's disease. These two disorders bear some striking similarities. Both cause chronic watery diarrhea, are more common
among Jewish people, and are rare in blacks and native Americans. Both exhibit a slight predominance in women, and the cause
of each disease is unknown, although an inappropriate immune

response is suspected. Both diseases carry an increased risk of intrinsic colon complications such as cancer, stricture, bleeding, perforation, and toxic megacolon. Also, both disorders may result in extracolonic complications such as iritis, arthritis, oral ulcers, erythema nodosum, and liver disease. However, it is important to differentiate between these two disorders because each has a different prognosis and treatment regimen.

Histologically, there are several differences between the two diseases. Ulcerative colitis consists of continuous involvement of the colon. The rectum is virtually always involved, and the terminal ileum usually is spared. Lesions consist of friable, bleeding microulcerations usually confined to the mucosa and submucosal tissues. The crypts of Lieberkühn are often involved. Crohn's disease, on the other hand, generally is not continuous, consisting of areas of normal tissue between areas of inflammation. The rectum usually is spared, and the terminal ileum is almost always affected. Crohn's lesions usually are linear ulcerations consisting of granulomas and fibrosis, which tend to be transmural.

The two conditions also have differing prognostic and therapeutic aspects. Crohn's disease tends to present more indolently. Patients may have minor symptoms of pain and nonbloody diarrhea for years before consulting a physician. Exacerbations and remissions of Crohn's disease are similarly slow and indolent, whereas those of ulcerative colitis tend to be much more dramatic. The complications of cancer and toxic megacolon are both less common in Crohn's disease than in ulcerative colitis. Medical therapy for both disorders consists of the use of antidiarrheal drugs, sulfasalazine, 5-acetylsalicylic acid preparations, and glucocorticoids, but initial response usually is more predictable in ulcerative colitis. Remissions are common in both disorders. If medical treatment fails, surgery is indicated for both diseases. Total proctocolectomy is curative for ulcerative colitis, but is only palliative for Crohn's disease.

ASSESSMENT

Mrs. S. is diagnosed with **ulcerative colitis** that is confirmed by colon biopsy. Her treatment plan may involve starting therapy with sulfasalazine or being referred to a gastroenterologist for care.

CASE 10-2

INITIAL PRESENTATION

A 67-year-old man presents with a chief complaint of abdominal pain and increasingly bulky, foul-smelling stools over the past 2 months. The patient states that he has been having four to five bowel movements a day. He reports that his stools tend to be oily and have a light, clay color. The stools tend to float, and it often takes two flushes to clear the toilet bowl. The abdominal pain is described as "gnawing and constant." It is generally epigastric but often radiates to the back. He also notes a 10-lb weight loss over the past 3 months, which he attributes to a loss of appetite. A careful review of systems reveals that his urine has been slightly darker than normal lately. The patient has a 38-pack-year history of smoking.

PHYSICAL EXAMINATION

The patient appears uncomfortable and worried. His conjunctiva are slightly icteric. His tongue and lips appear normal. An abdominal examination is significant for diffuse tenderness but is otherwise unremarkable with no organomegaly. The remainder of the physical examination is normal.

LABORATORY TESTS

Initial laboratory findings indicate slightly elevated levels of serum lipase and amylase as well as transaminases. In addition, alkaline phosphatase is increased to almost twice normal. The conjugated bilirubin is also increased. The CBC is within normal limits.

ASSESSMENT

This case involves chronic diarrhea but is notably different from the first in that there is an absence of blood in the stool. Large quantities of floating stool suggest increased fecal fat and thus raise concerns of fat malabsorption. Usually, this implies either a general problem in the small intestine (e.g., celiac sprue) or a pancreatic secretory dysfunction, which may be caused by a primary problem with the pancreas or a secondary hepatic or biliary problem that occludes secretion of pancreatic enzymes. Such diseases include pancreatitis, pancreatic cancer, primary biliary cirrhosis, hepatitis, cystic fibrosis, and carcinoma of the bile ducts. Generally, some diagnostic distinctions can be made between small intestinal pathology and pancreatic or biliary tract dysfunction. Weight loss due to anorexia and malabsorption usually is more prominent in those with intestinal disease, unless cancer has developed in the pancreas or biliary tract. Signs of vitamin deficiency, such as megaloblastic anemia, smooth tongue, or cheilosis, are much more common in patients with intestinal disorders.

Steatorrhea, however, is more prominent in patients with pancreatic or biliary diseases. In this case, the patient reports bulky, floating stools, which suggests steatorrhea. He also has no evidence of vitamin deficiency. He does have some additional signs, symptoms, and findings which alone suggest pancreatic involvement. Epigastric pain radiating to the back, for example, may be indicative of pancreatic disease. Dark urine, light stools, and icterus all indicate biliary obstruction, which results in decreased excretion of bilirubin into the gut and the corollary, increased blood levels of conjugated bilirubin. The laboratory findings confirm a conjugated hyperbilirubinemia compatible with an obstructive biliary problem. Because of the proximity of the pancreatic duct outlet to the common bile duct outlet, the exact nature of the obstructive problem is, at this point, unclear. Any pathologic process occluding the ampullae of Vater, for example, could produce these findings. A gallstone in the distal common bile duct or a tumor of the duct or adjacent tissues could cause obstruction and secondary elevations in serum bilirubin and pancreatic enzymes.

The insidious onset and progression of symptoms is ominous. First, the patient has an increased lipase level without severe pain. These factors indicate slowly progressive obstruction rather than acute pancreatitis. Second, the history of weight loss is disturbing. As noted above, pancreatic or biliary disease does not typically cause noticeable weight loss unless cancer is involved. Hepatitis and cholecystitis may cause the abnormal laboratory values seen here, but they do not usually cause weight loss. Finally, in addition to heart and lung disease, cigarette smoking is a risk factor for pancreatic carcinoma. This man has **obstructive biliary disease with pancreatic injury suggestive of tumor**. For these reasons, an abdominal computed tomography (CT) scan or the invasive but more accurate endoscopic retrograde cholangiopancreatography (ERCP) procedure would be a reasonable next step in this patient to evaluate for pancreatic cancer. The patient is referred to a gastroenterologist for this procedure.

CASE 10-3

INITIAL PRESENTATION

A 22-year-old woman presents with a chief complaint of diarrhea. For the past several years, she has been experiencing recurrent episodes of abdominal pain, bloating, and five to six episodes of watery diarrhea a day. She denies the presence of blood in her stools and states that they are of normal color. In addition, after meals she frequently experiences an urgency to defecate and minor abdominal pain during these episodes, which usually last for several days. The periods of diarrhea are usually followed by periods of constipation, which also lasts for several days before the cycle repeats itself. She states that episodes of diarrhea often are precipitated by emotional stress. She is concerned that this may be a serious medical problem. She has no other known health problems and takes no medications. She has no symptoms of hyperthyroidism. She has no history of travel or exposure to contaminated foods or water, and she denies any fevers or chills. Her family history is significant for anxiety disorders and depression on her mother's side. There is no family history of colon cancer.

PHYSICAL EXAMINATION

The patient is a young, well-nourished adult woman in no acute distress. Her skin, hair, and nails are normal. Her oropharynx is normal. Her abdomen is soft without tenderness to palpation. No masses or organomegaly are noted. A rectal examination is normal with a negative guaiac test. The remainder of the physical examination is within normal limits.

A CBC with differential, ESR, electrolytes, thyroid-stimulating hormone (TSH), and liver function tests all are within normal limits. A sigmoidoscopy is performed and also is unremarkable. Three stool samples are negative for occult blood.

This case presents some difficulties to the primary care physician largely in terms of treatment because there are no objective findings indicative of a pathologic process. In this instance, it might be helpful to reconsider the general causes of chronic diarrhea. So far in this chapter, there have been cases of inflammation (Case 10-1) and malabsorption (Case 10-2). Unlike those patients, this individual has no signs of such disorders. The absence of blood in her stool and any abnormal findings on sigmoidoscopy make an inflammatory process unlikely. Similarly, the absence of large, bulky stools; pancreatic or biliary symptoms; or vitamin deficiency is atypical for a malabsorptive disease. So what else could cause diarrhea? Increased secretions into the GI tract certainly can cause watery diarrhea, but this usually is the result of infection, and this patient has no risk factors or symptoms to suggest an infectious process. Without inflammation, hypersecretion, or malabsorption, increased GI motility is suspect. Increases in motility cause intestinal contents to move more quickly through the GI tract. As a result, absorption time is reduced. This may result in watery diarrhea. Diseases such as hyperthyroidism can cause increased GI motility, but in the absence of any such disorders, irritable bowel syndrome (IBS) is the most likely diagnosis.

IBS is probably the most common cause of chronic diarrhea in the United States, accounting for roughly half of the referrals to gastroenterologists and affecting more than 10% of the population. Patients often complain of alternating episodes of watery diarrhea and constipation, abdominal pain, and a feeling of bloating. There appears to be some relationship between this disorder and certain psychiatric problems, such as depression and anxiety.

ASSESSMENT

This patient has **IBS.** Her treatment plan includes asking her to keep a diary of food intake and bowel patterns to rule out a dietary intolerance. Referral for counseling is being considered.

Unfortunately, IBS is not only common, but it is also a disorder of exclusion. It is thought to be caused by an increase in the motility of the GI tract without an identifiable organic cause. Eating certain foods such as dairy products (as in lactose intolerance) may cause diarrhea similar to IBS. A careful history and a dietary record from the patient may help eliminate or confirm these possibilities. A workup should include tests for ESR, CBC, thyroid screen, and possibly liver function. The need for sigmoidoscopy is debatable. In a young patient with "typical" symptoms and no risk factors for serious organic disease, it is probably not cost-effective. Often the disorder can be treated effectively with antispasmodic agents and antidepressants. If, as in this case, the patient notes a clear association with levels of anxiety, counseling or other stress reduction techniques may be of value.

CASE 10-4

INITIAL PRESENTATION

A 38-year-old male accountant presents complaining of watery diarrhea and stomach cramps since yesterday, when the patient awoke with diffuse, cramping abdominal pain. Since then, he has had eight to ten episodes of watery diarrhea without blood. He has been able to drink fluids but has not felt like eating. He has had malaise and some slight nausea but denies vomiting. He denies recent travel or exposure to any known contaminants. He takes no medications and has no other medical illnesses.

PHYSICAL EXAMINATION

The patient appears ill and has a temperature of 100.4°F. His mucous membranes are moist, and his skin shows no rashes or tenting. His bowel sounds are hyperactive but of normal pitch. His abdomen is soft and slightly tender to palpation diffusely. No point tenderness or rebound tenderness is noted. No organomegaly or masses are detected. There are no other pertinent findings on physical examination.

ASSESSMENT

One of the most commonly used adages in medicine instructs physicians to think of horses, not zebras, when one hears hoofbeats. Often, clichés are clichés because they are worthy of being repeated. The acute nature of this patient's illness suggests an infectious etiology. Most cases of acute diarrhea are caused by infection by viral agents such as rotavirus, adenovirus, or Norwalk agent. These viruses are very common, and people often are not able to pinpoint any individuals around them who are sick. The infections are usually self-limited and last only 24–48 hours. Laboratory investigations usually are not helpful and unnecessary. As with other viral infections, care is supportive. In many cases, educating the patient about proper hand washing to prevent further spread of the disease is the most help a physician can give. In elderly or otherwise compromised patients, however, care should be taken to maintain water and electrolyte balance. Such patients are at higher risk for dehydration.

This man has **viral or food poisoning gastroenteritis.** As a cause of acute gastroenteritis, food poisoning may be even more common than intestinal viral infections, and the two may be clinically indistinguishable. It is worth asking if others who have eaten the same food became ill. There are no readily available tests to confirm the presence of a viral infection or a foodborne toxin, but because the treatment for both illnesses is supportive, the lack of a firm diagnosis is not a significant problem. In cases of food poisoning, nausea and vomiting are the prominent symptoms, in viral illnesses, diarrhea may be the dominant symptom.

Suppression of diarrhea (or vomiting for that matter) in gastroenteritis of any cause is not wise during the first 48 hours of the illness. Vomiting and diarrhea help rid the intestinal tract of toxins and, thus, when these symptoms are eliminated, the illness may be prolonged. The patient should drink fluids to avoid dehydration. If the fever persists or if abdominal pain increases or hydration cannot be maintained, he should seek further medical attention.

CASE 10-5

INITIAL PRESENTATION

A 19-year-old woman presents complaining of diarrhea. She reports that she has experienced watery diarrhea, stomach cramps, and two episodes of vomiting for the past several days since returning from a 2-day field trip with an anthropology class to an undeveloped region. The patient complains also of chills, malaise, and nausea. She tells you that she brought her own water but ate the local foods. The remainder of her medical history is unremarkable.

PHYSICAL EXAMINATION

The patient is a well-nourished woman who appears slightly ill. She has a temperature of 101°F. Her mucous membranes are moist, and there is no skin tenting. The abdomen is diffusely tender to palpation but is otherwise normal. There are no other abnormalities on physical examination.

ASSESSMENT

Note that this case is very similar to Case 10-4. This patient has an acute diarrheal illness with stomach cramps, malaise, and nausea. As in Case 10-4, the nature of her symptoms suggests an infectious etiology. However, this patient's travel history is clearly an additional risk factor. Travel to less developed areas of the world or exposure to contaminated food or water commonly causes **"traveler's diarrhea."** Typically, this is a self-limited diarrheal illness that begins within a few days of exposure. In rare cases, the disease can be serious. Not drinking the water is wise when traveling in such areas. However, ingestion of undercooked food may be a more likely source of contaminants. *Escherichia coli* is by far the most common cause, with *Shigella* being the second most common. Usually, there is no need for in-depth laboratory evaluation, and supportive care is all that is required. However, if the disease is prolonged or severe, further investigations, including stool culture, may be necessary. Chemoprophylactic regimens are available to individuals who are planning travel to endemic areas. Unfortunately, antibiotic use is yet another cause of acute diarrhea.

CASE 10-6

INITIAL PRESENTATION

A 39-year-old homosexual man presents complaining of diarrhea. His symptoms began roughly 10 days ago with the onset of abdominal cramps, nausea, and profuse watery diarrhea. At the time, the patient felt he had "the flu." These symptoms resolved within 1 week, but the patient then began experiencing fever; tenesmus; and bloody, mucoid diarrhea. The patient has no other medical problems and takes no medications.

PHYSICAL EXAMINATION

The patient is a middle-aged man who appears acutely ill. His temperature is 101°F. His heart and lungs are clear. Bowel sounds are present, somewhat hyperactive, and of normal pitch. Abdominal examination is significant for some mild diffuse tenderness but is otherwise unremarkable. There are no other abnormalities on physical examination. A stool culture is positive for *Shigella flexneri*.

ASSESSMENT

Shigella is one of the many bacterial agents that commonly infect the GI tract. Others include *Campylobacter, E. coli, Klebsiella, Serratia, Salmonella, Citrobacter, Proteus,* and *Yersinia* species. Parasitic infections such as *Giardia lamblia* and *Entamoeba histolytica* also can cause acute diarrhea and should be suspected when patients have visited endemic areas. *Shigella* infection is most common in children, homosexual men, persons traveling to lesser developed countries, and people confined to institutions. Typically, the bacteria initially attack the small intestine, producing cramping and often voluminous watery diarrhea. Within a few days, the bacteria localize to the colon, where they invade the mucosa causing bloody, mucoid diarrhea. Fortunately, the disease is generally self-limited and resolves within 1–4 weeks. One major exception to this rule is *Shigella dysenteriae*, which can be fatal even in previously healthy adults.

There are two major points in this case that are important to clinical problem-solving. The first is that he is a homosexual man. As discussed throughout this book, individuals are at differing risks for certain pathologies based on risk factors such as age, ethnicity, work and living environment, and life style. Awareness of a patient's risk factors can reduce time to diagnosis and facilitate good patient care. The second aspect of this case that makes it different from others addressed thus far is the presence of acute bloody diarrhea. As previously discussed, most cases of acute diarrhea are infectious and self-limited. In most of these cases, extensive laboratory investigation is neither necessary nor effective. However, the presence of blood in the stool suggests tissue damage, and bacterial stool culture is recommended because this is the only definitive diagnosis for most enterotoxic bacteria. Stool culture usually is both specific and sensitive. However, roughly half of the patients with acute bloody diarrhea have negative cultures.

In patients with *Shigella*, antibiotic treatment is suggested to shorten the course of the disease and to decrease excretion of organisms. However, resistance does develop via plasmid transfer. Therefore, antibiotic treatment varies throughout different areas of the world. As with other enteric infections, fluid and electrolyte balance should be maintained. If diarrhea is not profuse, this can usually be done orally. This man is diagnosed with ***Shigella* enteritis,** and he should begin trimethoprim/sulfamethoxazole pending antibiotic-sensitivity results. The patient should be advised to maintain hydration and should be educated regarding risk factors for *Shigella* enteritis.

CASE 10-7

INITIAL PRESENTATION

A 56-year-old man who is a former construction worker complains of constipation. The patient states that he has had less than one bowel movement every 2 days for the past several weeks. He also notes an associated feeling of bloating. He denies any other symptoms and has never experienced this before. He is currently on workers' compensation because of a back injury he suffered 8 weeks ago at a construction site. He has been taking propoxyphene on a regular basis for back and lower extremity pain ever since the accident. Otherwise, he has no medical problems and takes no medications. He has never had any hospitalizations or surgeries.

PHYSICAL EXAMINATION

The physical examination is significant for some stiffness in the lower back but is otherwise unremarkable.

ASSESSMENT

Like diarrhea, constipation is defined differently by different people. What is normal for one person may be constipation for another. This is not to say that bowel habits that are "normal" or usual for an individual are not a risk factor. People with less frequent bowel movements have a higher incidence of colon cancer. When the bowel movements are not grossly abnormal, a significant change in the pattern may be more important.

Unlike diarrhea, constipation usually is not the result of infectious pathologies. Constipation is frequently idiopathic, particularly among the elderly. However, it is important to try to rule out any underlying cause initially. Common causes of constipation include hypothyroidism, depression, and autonomic neuropathy. All of these conditions cause hypomotility of the intestinal tract. Inadequate fluid intake may result in hard stools that are passed infrequently and sometimes with significant discomfort. Finally, intestinal obstruction may cause constipation but usually with other symptoms and signs such as abdominal distention, blood in the stools, and high-pitched bowel sounds.

In a patient without underlying medical conditions, associated symptoms, or history of surgery, a primary medical condition is less likely. In this case, one of the most significant factors in the patient's history is medication use. Constipation is one of the most common complaints of patients on pain control therapy. All of the narcotic analgesics potentially can cause constipation. This can present problems with chronic pain control but is usually limited to an uncomfortable side effect. Occasionally, however, fecal impaction can occur, creating the need for further medical (and sometimes surgical) intervention.

This patient is diagnosed with **constipation as a result of medication use.** The treatment plan for a patient with constipation from a medication is to first switch to a nonconstipating drug such as ibuprofen or acetaminophen. If these do not control the pain then a return to a more potent but constipating drug may be necessary along with a regimen to treat the constipation. Bowel stimulants such as bisacodyl and a high-fiber diet with plenty of fluids may sufficiently counteract the effects of the pain medication.

SUMMARY

Chronic diarrhea can be divided into various categories based on pathology and presentation. Clinically, it is helpful to determine the type of diarrhea initially. Bloody diarrhea is indicative of damage to the GI mucosa. Inflammatory bowel disease, cancer, hemorrhoids, tissue-toxic medications, and radiation exposure all can induce tissue damage. Each of these etiologies can best be investigated via assessment of associated symptoms and risk factors. Chronic diarrhea consisting of bulky, floating stools is indicative of a malabsorption problem. In general, such a problem is the result of either an inability to excrete pancreatic enzymes necessary for digestion properly into the GI tract or an inability to absorb GI contents due to an anatomic or physiologic problem of the small intestine. Differentiation among these etiologies often is straightforward.

Intestinal dysfunction usually results in more prominent vitamin deficiency and weight loss, whereas pancreatic enzyme problems are more likely to result in steatorrhea. If doubt still remains, a variety of biochemical indicators can be used to confirm a diagnosis. Watery diarrhea results from either excessive intestinal secretions or increased GI motility that does not allow adequate time for water absorption. Increased secretions usually result from infection, which is not a typical cause of chronic diarrhea. Irritable bowel syndrome, causing increased motility, is an extremely common cause of chronic watery diarrhea. However, other causes (e.g., hyperthyroidism, antibiotic use, laxative abuse) must be ruled out. Previous gastric or bowel surgery also may cause chronic diarrhea if regions of the GI tract that are critical for absorption of nutrients or water have been resected.

Acute diarrhea, although very common, is usually self-limited. Most often, the disorder is caused by infection from viruses, bacteria, or parasites, and the symptomatology of each of these etiologies is often very similar. Laboratory evaluation is often unnecessary. The exceptions to this are cases in which diarrhea becomes chronic or severe, blood is present in the stool, or certain risk factors, such as general debilitation, are associated with the disease. When stool culture is performed, and a definitive diagnosis is made, antibiotic treatment often is effective in limiting the course of the disease. Maintenance of fluid and electrolyte balance is important and can be done orally or intravenously, depending on the severity of the diarrhea.

In cases of acute diarrhea in which an infectious etiology can be excluded, other causes such as acute anxiety, hyperthyroidism, and medication use (particularly antibiotics) should be considered.

Constipation is usually due to decreased motility of the bowel, inadequate fluid intake causing hard stools, inadequate fiber intake to stimulate bowel activity, or an obstruction. Hypomotility may be secondary to medications, intrinsic autonomic neuropathy, especially in the elderly, or a systemic condition such as hypothyroidism or depression. Obstruction is occasionally the result of one of the other causes, which has progressed too far, but most often obstruction is from adhesions from previous surgery or from a tumor of the bowel. Treatment must be directed at the cause. If it is possible to change precipitating factors, then this should be done. If a medication is indicated, then the type of drug should be chosen on the basis of the cause. An example would be the use of a stimulant to treat decreased motility for which the cause cannot be eliminated.

CHAPTER 11
Chief Complaint: Frequent Urination

CASE 11-1

INITIAL PRESENTATION

Mrs. A., a 36-year-old high school teacher, presents with a complaint of frequent urination. She states that she normally urinates every few hours but now is urinating roughly once an hour. She also is getting up at least twice during the night to urinate. She finds it difficult to get through an entire lecture without excusing herself to use the bathroom. She notes no dysuria, color changes, or discharge. Upon further questioning, the patient admits to accompanying increased thirst. These symptoms began roughly 2–3 months ago and have been getting progressively worse. She reports a slight lack of energy over the same time period but otherwise has no complaints. She never has had any other medical problems other than being overweight her entire adult life. However, she states that she has actually managed to lose about 5 lbs over the past month "without even trying." Mrs. A. takes no medications other than an occasional aspirin for minor aches and pains. She has no allergies to any medications of which she is aware. She does not see a physician on a regular basis because she "has always been healthy." Mrs. A. lives with her husband and two children. Her family history is significant for both parents having adult-onset diabetes mellitus (type 2 DM).

> No associated urinary symptoms

> Associated increased thirst

PHYSICAL EXAMINATION

Mrs. A. weighs 204 lbs; her height is 64 inches. Her blood pressure is 138/86 mm Hg, her pulse is 84 beats/min, and her respirations are 16 breaths/min. Mrs. A. appears to be a pleasant, overweight woman in no distress.

Her skin has normal turgor; no lesions are noted. A head, eyes, ears, nose, and throat (HEENT) examination is unremarkable. Her mucous membranes are moist. The fundi appear normal. Her neck is supple without masses or lymphadenopathy. There are no carotid bruits. No masses or discharge are noted in her breasts. Her lungs are clear to percussion and auscultation. A cardiac examination reveals a regular rate without murmurs, gallops, or rubs. Her abdomen is obese, soft, and nontender with no organomegaly. No abnormalities are noted in her extremities. The remainder of the physical examination is unremarkable.

1. What are the basic causes of increased urine production?

Discussion

In other chapters of this book, the value of categorizing patients' problems is discussed. By ruling in or out broad categories, one often can narrow a list of hypotheses in relatively few steps. In this case, it is helpful to understand the general causes of polyuria and differentiate among them. One of the most basic functions of the kidneys is to regulate the osmolality of the blood and the overall volume of fluid in the body. Basically, if the body is overhydrated, and osmolality is therefore low, the kidneys respond by increasing the volume of urine produced. If, on the other hand, the body is dehydrated, urine is concentrated, and volume is reduced. Therefore, a disturbance in either fluid volume or osmolality can result in an increase in urine production. (Other "perceived" causes of increased urination are discussed later in this chapter.)

2. What risk factors does this patient have that might suggest a disorder that could explain her frequent urination?

Diabetes mellitus (DM) is discussed in several chapters of this book. It is an extremely important disease to consider in internal medicine because it is so prevalent, it can have serious complications, and it often can be controlled with proper recognition and appropriate therapy. Interestingly, although the term "diabetes" is used commonly to refer to DM, the term actually refers to a diverse group of diseases characterized by increased urination. This patient has several indications of possible DM.

1. The patient has been overweight for most of her adult life. It is often helpful to think in terms of risk factors both for diagnostic and preventive reasons. In other words, physicians must not merely think of what patients have but also for what they are at risk. This is extremely important for determining the meaning of positive laboratory tests

and for preventing patients from having serious diseases. Obesity is prevalent in the adult American population. It puts people at risk for a variety of disorders, including DM.

2. This patient has recently lost some weight "without trying." DM is a state in which the body is either deprived of insulin or is incapable of using it. In either case, the effects of insulin are lacking. As a result, cells are deprived of sugar. In adipose tissue, fats are broken down to provide energy because glucose is relatively unavailable. Muscle tissue is unable to use glucose for glycogenesis or protein synthesis. In simple (but ultimately realistic) terms, the body starves, and weight loss occurs.

3. Lack of energy also is a consistent finding in patients with DM. Excessive thirst (polydipsia) is not unique to DM, but it often occurs with any osmotic diuresis.

4. The most significant risk factor for DM in this patient is her family history. Type 2 DM, or noninsulin-dependent DM, clearly has a genetic component, and patients with two diabetic parents should be considered at high risk for the disease.

3. What laboratory tests might help to define the problem further?

If DM is suspected, a physician may take a variety of next steps. A fasting glucose level is somewhat helpful for confirmation. However, serum glucose levels often fluctuate rapidly. A hemoglobin A_{1c} (HbA_{1c}) test measures the glycosylation of hemoglobin; therefore, this test is a good indicator of the overall levels of blood sugar during the life span of a red blood cell (RBC), or approximately 120 days. Evidence of a chronically elevated blood glucose is a better indicator of DM than a series of single measurements. This is not to say that single blood glucose levels are not important. They may or may not reflect DM, but they certainly demand an explanation.

LABORATORY TESTS

A number of laboratory tests were ordered for this patient. A complete blood count (CBC) and sequential multiple analysis with seven different tests (SMA-7) are within normal limits, except for a fasting blood glucose level of 162 mg/dL. Her HbA_{1c} is 10.4% (normal = 4.0%–7.0%). Urinalysis shows 3+ glucose but is otherwise normal.

4. What long-term problems pose a risk for this patient?

Discussion

The importance of understanding risk factors cannot be stressed enough. Diabetic patients are at risk for cardiovascular disease, nephropathy, retinopathy, microvascular problems, neuropathy, and other probable autoimmune disorders, such as hypothyroidism. As a result, diabetic patients should be taught to keep their feet clean and dry to make infection less likely. They must check their feet regularly for signs of infection that otherwise may not be noticed because of neurologic dysfunction that may diminish sensation. Diabetics should be screened for hypertension and hyperlipidemia. Also, they should undergo annual ophthalmologic examinations for any signs of retinopathy. Finally, patients with diabetes should have their urine checked for protein. It is important to be aware that a simple urinalysis is not sensitive enough to detect early proteinuria. Diabetic patients should have either a 24-hour urine test or a morning spot microalbumin test at least once a year. A positive microalbumin test indicates the onset of diabetic renal disease, and starting these patients on an angiotensin-converting enzyme (ACE) inhibitor substantially retards or prevents the development of renal failure. These patients need an ACE inhibitor even if they do not have hypertension.

5. What causes polyuria in patients with DM?

Polyuria may be a sign of an osmotic diuresis. Causes of increased urination often can loosely be categorized into volume overload and osmotic imbalance. Uncontrolled DM is one of many hyperosmotic states. Any disorder that increases osmotic particles in the serum can have the same results. This category includes hyperglycemia and hypercalcemia caused by hyperparathyroidism or neoplasms that have metastasized to bone. When serum osmolality is increased by a relative increase in solute that can be filtered or secreted into the urine, such a solute draws water along with it. As a result, urine volume (and therefore output) is increased. This is known as an osmotic diuresis. Many substances can increase the osmolality of body fluids. However, electrolytes (particularly sodium), urea, and glucose are the major factors in most cases. Plasma osmolality (P_{osm}) can be approximated using the following equation:

$$P_{osm} = 2 \times [Na^+] + ([Glucose]/18) + ([BUN]/2.8)$$

Urea is a relatively ineffective osmole, and because the concentration of glucose is much lower than sodium, the glucose and blood urea nitrogen (BUN) portions of this equation often are overlooked. However, in this case, glucose concentrations may be greatly elevated (an HbA_{1c} of 10.4% is roughly equivalent to an average serum glucose of 180 mg/dL); thus, glucose levels cannot be ignored. The patient is frequently thirsty because she is losing excess water in her urine.

ASSESSMENT

Mrs. A. is diagnosed with **type 2 DM.** Her treatment plan includes extensive DM education, as well as a diet, exercise, and weight-loss program.

CASE 11-2

INITIAL PRESENTATION

A 77-year-old woman with a history of coronary artery disease (CAD) and congestive heart failure (CHF) complains of progressively worsening nocturia during the past month. She used to sleep through the night but is now getting up 2–3 times per night to urinate. She states that she does not notice frequent urination so much during the day. The patient also has noted increased swelling in her lower extremities over the past several weeks. She takes lovastatin for high cholesterol, digoxin for "heart problems," and nitroglycerin tablets as needed for angina. She states that she has not had any chest pain in several years and that she has not been able to refill her medications lately because of money problems. She says she has been cutting her medication dosage in half over the past few weeks to compensate.

PHYSICAL EXAMINATION

The physical examination is significant for a 10-lb weight gain since her last visit 6 months ago, a soft third heart sound (S_3) gallop, and 2+ pitting pedal edema, but is otherwise unremarkable.

Increased urine output may be caused by osmotic disturbances or volume overload. This is an example of the latter. An S_3 gallop is indicative of turbulent filling of the ventricles, usually caused by volume overload. The weight gain experienced by this patient also may be an indication of fluid retention.

6. What is the mechanism that causes water retention in a
   patient with cardiac failure?

Discussion

Heart failure provides a very interesting case study of kidney function in terms of volume regulation. It is noteworthy that this patient does not complain of polyuria during the day. When she is not supine, the blood vessels in the lower extremities are distended due to increased pressure of gravity on the "column" of blood in the body. As a result, blood tends to pool in the lower extremities, and venous return to the heart is decreased. An individual with a healthy heart compensates for this decreased venous return by increasing heart rate and stroke volume to maintain cardiac output. However, a patient with CHF has a diminished capacity to increase cardiac output as needed. As a result, more blood remains in the venous side, and the increased pressure eventually causes pedal edema as well as congestion in the liver and spleen (backward failure). On the arterial side, diminished cardiac output causes decreased perfusion of peripheral tissues, including the kidneys (forward failure). At this point, the total amount of water in the body is unchanged, but the volume is redistributed toward the venous side. Unfortunately, the kidneys remain "unaware" of this fact. This is an interesting example of how organs in the body function in many cases as individual entities. From the kidneys' "point of view," the body is dehydrated. The juxtaglomerular apparatus has no way of knowing where the volume of blood has gone; it only knows that the kidneys are not being adequately perfused. The kidneys respond by producing renin, which converts angiotensinogen to angiotensin I, which is subsequently converted to angiotensin II by ACE in the lungs. Angiotensin II stimulates aldosterone production by the zona glomerulosa of the adrenal cortex. Aldosterone, in turn, stimulates the reabsorption of sodium and water in exchange for hydrogen and potassium in the distal convoluted tubule of the kidney.

Although somewhat drawn out, this pathway is fundamental to understanding volume regulation. The bottom line is that the lack of renal perfusion caused by poor cardiac output results in water retention by the kidneys. This partially explains why this patient has an S_3 gallop and does not complain of increased urination during the day. At night, however, the situation is reversed. When the body is supine, gravity no longer affects a large column of blood that can distend the vessels of the lower extremities. Instead, venous blood is distributed relatively evenly throughout the body, and blood flow back to the heart is not impeded. Because cardiac output can be maintained in this position, the kidneys can be fully perfused. Now, the body attempts to compensate for the increased volume of water taken on during the day. Renin production is inhibited, eventually resulting in a decrease in aldosterone production and a subsequent diminution of sodium and water reabsorption. If the imbalance from inadequate cardiac output is mild enough, all edema fluid is reabsorbed while the patient is recumbent. As the situation progresses, the excess tissue fluid takes longer to return to the circulatory system, and a more continuously edematous state results.

Other factors such as antidiuretic hormone (ADH), tissue elasticity, serum proteins, and "third space" effects all may play a role in fluid balance and fluid shifts. These processes, however, are of secondary importance to the physiologic response of the kidneys to decreased cardiac output as described above.

ASSESSMENT

This patient has all of the signs, symptoms, and risk factors for **worsening CHF due to a reduction in medication.** She has nocturia, ankle edema, a history of CHF, an S_3 gallop, a 10-lb weight gain, and a history of noncompliance. Most likely, this patient's heart failure was managed with her previous dose of digoxin, but it is not being managed on the reduced dose. All of the medications taken by this patient, with the exception of nitroglycerin, have relatively long-lasting effects, which often are not well understood by patients. These types of medications are likely the first to be discontinued when patients have difficulty with side effects or money. It is very important to explain fully to patients the reason for taking their medications and the potential consequences if these medications are discontinued. Additionally, there are a variety of means available to help patients pay for medications that should be explored by both the physician and the patient.

CASE 11-3

INITIAL PRESENTATION

A 24-year-old man is brought to the emergency department after falling in a bicycle race. He has a head wound and a broken ankle. Radiographs show no evidence of a skull fracture. His ankle is placed in a cast, and his lacerations and abrasions are treated. He is told he suffered a concussion head injury and is sent home to rest.

Two days later, he presents in the clinic complaining of excessive thirst and frequent urination. The patient states that until now, he has been in excellent health. He exercises regularly, takes no medications on a regular basis, and does not drink, smoke, or use drugs. He has never experienced these symptoms before.

PHYSICAL EXAMINATION

The patient is alert and oriented to person, place, and time. His head and left ankle are bandaged. He has some periorbital edema, bilaterally. His funduscopic examination shows no evidence of papilledema.

LABORATORY TESTS

The results of laboratory tests ordered on admission are given below.

Laboratory Tests	Patient	Normal Values
Sodium (Na$^+$)	145 mEq/L	136–146 mEq/L
Potassium (K$^+$)	4.8 mEq/L	3.5–5.1 mEq/L
Chloride (Cl$^-$)	106 mEq/L	98–106 mEq/L
Blood urea nitrogen (BUN)	16 mg/dL	7–18 mg/dL
Creatinine	1.2 mg/dL	0.7–1.3 mg/dL
White blood cells (WBC)	6200 cells/mm^3	4500–11,000 cells/mm^3
Hemoglobin	17 g/dL	13.5–17.5 g/dL
Hematocrit	49%	39%–49%
Urinalysis	Specific gravity = 1.002	1.000–1.030 sp gr

ASSESSMENT

Taken individually, all of these laboratory values are within normal limits. However, general trends often are just as important as specific figures. Virtually all of the laboratory measurements of the serum are at the upper end of normal. Taken individually, this could indicate an increase in a particular factor such as too much sodium in the body. However, it would be unlikely that the absolute amounts of all of these substances are increased. A more plausible hypothesis is that each is increased "artificially" due to a concentration effect. In other words, if the total amount of free water in the body were decreased (as in a dehydration state), then each of the measured factors would be concentrated in the serum and appear to be above normal. Of course, the reverse also would be true if there were too much free water in the serum. The question then becomes: Where did all of the free water go? This patient's history indicates that he is urinating frequently. In addition, the specific gravity of the urine indicates that it is quite dilute. Then, the free water must have gone into the urine. The next obvious question is: Why did the free water "shift" from the serum to the urine? The role of aldosterone was discussed in Case 11-2. Here, the situation is significantly different. Unlike Case 11-2 in which water was drawn into the urine following sodium, in this case, free water is apparently being excreted. This suggests an ADH disturbance. ADH increases permeability of the collecting duct to water. The concentrated environment of the renal medulla, created by the countercurrent exchange mechanism of the loop of Henle, sets up an osmotic gradient that pulls water out of the collecting duct in the presence of ADH. However, in the absence of ADH, the collecting duct is relatively impermeable to water. Despite the osmotic gradient, water remains in the duct, eventually being excreted in the urine.

ADH is a polypeptide hormone produced in the posterior pituitary gland. When the pituitary gland is injured (as might occur with a head injury), ADH production may be compromised. Typically, cases such as this present with polyuria and polydipsia for a period of 4–5 days. During this time, the dysfunctional pituitary gland is unable to release ADH, which therefore remains in the neurohypophysis. This period is often followed by the release of the stored ADH, causing the reverse condition. Most notably, severe hyponatremia may result. After another 4–5 days, ADH levels again diminish as the stored ADH is depleted. If the pituitary gland is sufficiently damaged, this final phase may be permanent, resulting in chronic ADH deficiency. The condition is known as central diabetes insipidus. The term "central" distinguishes this disorder from nephrogenic diabetes insipidus, in which the kidneys are not responsive to ADH. In other cases, the onset pattern or presentation of symptoms is discussed in relation to the diagnosis. The sudden onset of this patient's symptoms following his accident should arouse suspicion of a traumatic injury-related problem.

The test results suggest that the kidneys are not responding appropriately to the concentration of serum electrolytes. The high-normal serum sodium level should cause the kidneys to elaborate a concentrated urine and thus retain free water. Instead, there is a dilute urine with a low specific gravity. A simultaneous serum and urine osmolality would confirm or reject the hypothesis of an inappropriate renal response to a free water imbalance. If the osmolalities are indeed abnormal, exogenous ADH could be given to see if this corrects the problem. No change after exogenous ADH indicates renal insensitivity to ADH, which is a very unlikely possibility given the acute onset of the problem following head trauma. An imaging study of the pituitary gland, such as magnetic resonance imaging (MRI), would further delineate structural damage to the gland.

This man is diagnosed with **probable acute central diabetes insipidus secondary to head trauma.** It is possible that he may have permanent central diabetes insipidus. The patient's fluid and electrolyte balance should be followed carefully through the acute phase then evaluated for chronic central diabetes insipidus as described above. An MRI of his pituitary gland will be performed.

CASE 11-4

INITIAL PRESENTATION

A 32-year-old woman presents complaining of frequent urination. She states her symptoms began yesterday morning and have been getting progressively worse. She has a constant sense of urinary urgency. She has been urinating almost every hour; however, the volume of urine is smaller than normal. She also notes some discomfort in the urethral region when urinating. Slight chills have been present over the past few hours.

PHYSICAL EXAMINATION

The physical examination is normal except for a temperature of 101.2°F and slight suprapubic tenderness.

ASSESSMENT

It is questionable whether this patient is actually having an increased urine output as the other patients had. Although she notes increased frequency of urination, she also notes decreased urine volume. In addition, she describes some associated urinary symptoms in the form of urgency and dysuria. Also, the progressively worsening nature of her symptoms and associated chills and fever suggest an infectious etiology. Urinary bladder infections are more common in women. Other risk factors include pregnancy, previous urinary tract infection, and DM. A urinalysis for this patient would most likely reveal evidence of a bacterial infection, and the diagnosis would be **urinary tract infection.** In this case, the patient should be started on an appropriate antibiotic such as trimethoprim/sulfamethoxazole until urine culture and sensitivity results are returned.

CASE 11-5

INITIAL PRESENTATION

A 62-year-old man presents with a chief complaint of increasingly frequent urination over the past year. He states that he usually needs to urinate at least once per hour and gets up at least three times each night. He notes no pain on urination, no fever or chills, and no changes in urine color or odor. The man tells you that the volume of urine is usually small, and he frequently feels as if his bladder is not fully emptied after urinating. He needs to strain to initiate a stream of urine. He starts and stops several times when urinating. The man is otherwise healthy and takes no medications. He has no significant family history.

PHYSICAL EXAMINATION

The patient is a well-nourished man who appears his stated age and is in no apparent distress. A HEENT examination is unremarkable. His neck is supple and reveals no bruits or lymphadenopathy. His chest is clear to percussion and auscultation. His heart is beating at a regular rate with no murmurs and no S_3 or S_4. His abdomen is soft and nontender. No lesions, cyanosis, or edema are noted in his extremities. Pulses are 2+ bilaterally in upper and lower extremities. He has a normal, circumcised penis; his testes are descended bilaterally, and there are no masses. His prostate gland is enlarged and smooth without notable masses or tenderness. A guaiac test is negative. Urinalysis is normal and shows no traces of blood.

ASSESSMENT

This case bears similarities to others presented in this chapter. As in the case of the woman with a urinary tract infection (Case 11-4), this patient is noting frequent urination but with smaller volumes of urine. There is no indication that the overall amount of urine production is increased as in Cases 11-1 and 11-2. Unlike Case 11-4, however, this patient exhibits no signs of infection. The slow, progressive nature of this patient's disease suggests a degenerative process as seen in the case of Mrs. A. (Case 11-1). This man's symptoms suggest that he has a partial obstruction of his urinary tract. Benign prostatic hyperplasia (BPH) is extremely common in elderly men and should be suspected when a man older than 50 years complains of frequent urination and obstructive symptoms such as the need to strain to urinate, difficulty maintaining the stream, and the inability to completely empty the bladder. Some estimates suggest that the percent of men older than 50 years having some degree of BPH is roughly equal to their age. Thus, 60% of men 60 years of age and 70% of men 70 years of age and so on have BPH. The diagnosis is generally confirmed by the finding of a nontender, smooth, enlarged prostate on physical examination. The symptoms are usually straightforward, and the diagnosis is made clinically. A urinalysis can rule out signs of infection or bleeding. Of course, the major concern is not to overlook a possible neoplasm. Further investigation is not necessary unless there are signs of prostate cancer (e.g., nodularity, hematuria). Currently, there is still debate over the usefulness of a prostate-specific antigen (PSA) blood test. Although the antibody is usually increased in men with prostate cancer, it also may be elevated in those with BPH. The high incidence of false-positive PSA results may lead to unnecessary further testing, which is both expensive and invasive. Biopsy is definitive, and newer ultrasound techniques appear promising. If a PSA test is performed, a rising level from year to year appears to be more specific for prostate cancer than simply an elevated titer. In addition, recent studies have refixed the normal values for PSA and further improved the specificity of the test.

This patient is diagnosed with **BPH.** His treatment plan is to begin a regimen of α-adrenergic blocker medication. In the past, surgery was the only available treatment for BPH. More recently, 5α-reductase inhibitors have been used to shrink the prostate, but the long-term cost–benefit ratio has been seriously questioned. α-Adrenergic blockers are quite effective in reducing symptoms quickly and are currently the treatment of choice. Any "mechanical" disorder that interferes with complete emptying of the bladder can result in frequent urination. If the bladder cannot be fully emptied, the bladder quickly becomes full. Neurologic, muscular, and other obstructive diseases, therefore, all can cause frequent urination.

CASE 11-6

INITIAL PRESENTATION

A 54-year-old woman complains of increasing nocturia over the past several months. The patient also notes increased thirst over the same time period and feels that her total urine output has increased. She is a regular patient of the internal medicine clinic. She has suffered from chronic back problems after a motor vehicle

accident 22 years ago for which she takes aspirin and acetaminophen daily. She has suffered in the past from recurrent gastritis and
normocytic anemia. Currently, she denies fever or chills and does
not suffer from any other known medical problems.

PHYSICAL EXAMINATION

The patient's vital signs are as follows: temperature is normal;
pulse, 96 beats/min; and blood pressure, 108/64 mm Hg. Her
mucous membranes are dry. The remainder of the physical examination is unremarkable.

LABORATORY TESTS

A CBC is normal except for a slight normocytic anemia. BUN and
creatinine levels are both slightly increased in equal proportions.
Urinalysis reveals a dilute urine that is positive for protein, WBCs,
and RBCs, but negative for glucose.

ASSESSMENT

This case is similar to that of Mrs. A. in Case 11-1, who suffered
from DM, in that both patients note increased overall urine output.
In addition, both individuals had polydipsia. This patient also has
signs of dehydration on physical examination. One significant difference in this case from the others is the elevated BUN and creatinine levels. One might expect these to be increased in any patient
with dehydration, but because urea nitrogen usually can be reabsorbed in the nephron, the ratio of BUN to creatinine would be
increased in a case of significant dehydration. The increased BUN
and creatinine levels, in addition to the findings of protein, WBCs,
and RBCs in the urine, raise the concern of kidney involvement.
Many chronic diseases suppress erythropoiesis. In addition, dis-
eased kidneys produce less erythropoietin. The normocytic anemia
also is consistent with prolonged kidney dysfunction. Although
there are WBCs in the urine, there are no other signs of possible
infection, and the chronic nature of her symptoms suggests a
degenerative, immunologic, neoplastic, or other relatively slowly
progressing pathology. There are a great number of kidney disorders. Often intensive laboratory investigation is required for diagnosis. In other cases, the history can provide important clues. In
patients with chronic illnesses such as DM or systemic lupus
erythematosus (SLE), for example, renal involvement is common
and even anticipated.

This woman has only one fairly significant current medical condition: chronic back pain. She also has a history of gastritis and
anemia. It is difficult to make a connection between a traumatic
event that occurred many years ago and current kidney problems.

However, there may be a connection between the medications she is presently taking and her renal dysfunction. One possibility in this case would be **drug-induced chronic interstitial nephritis.** This disorder is more common in women, and it typically occurs in patients with chronic headaches, backaches, or arthritic disorders who chronically use high doses of analgesics. The disorder was first described following phenacetin use, but analgesics containing aspirin, caffeine, and acetaminophen also have been associated with the disorder. It is theorized that metabolites of phenacetin (such as acetaminophen) directly damage the renal tubules. Aspirin may potentiate damage by inhibiting vasodilating prostaglandins, resulting in ischemia. Sterile pyuria is extremely common, and, initially, patients are often unable to concentrate their urine. The anemia common to many renal diseases may be exacerbated by RBC destruction by drug metabolites. Renal impairment is progressive and can result in end-stage renal disease (ESRD) if left unchecked. Fortunately, with cessation of analgesic use, adequate hydration, and, if present, control of hypertension, progressive renal impairment usually can be halted and occasionally slightly reversed. Finally, her previous gastritis may have been caused by analgesic use. And, blood loss from the irritated stomach may have contributed to the anemia.

SUMMARY

As with other symptoms presented to internists, a comprehensive history is the first step in diagnosis. Frequent urination may or may not indicate increased urine output. In cases of normal urine output, associated symptoms and a thorough risk factor assessment usually distinguish between a mechanical or infectious etiology. When an unexplained diuresis occurs, osmotic or volume disturbances, medications, or renal dysfunction are suspect. Again, a thorough history usually is the most productive, cost-effective diagnostic tool. An intravenous pyelogram, imaging study, or even a biopsy may be necessary to confirm a diagnosis, but a simple, inexpensive urinalysis may provide critical initial information.

Throughout this book, cases that are typical and educational have been presented. It should be noted that chronic interstitial nephritis (Case 11-6) is not common and is not likely to be one's first diagnostic impression. It was presented here to illustrate three important points. First, this case illustrated the importance of medication involvement. Drug-induced chronic interstitial nephritis often may be difficult to diagnose because patients may not consider over-the-counter drugs as "medications" and may not report chronic use. Second, this case once again illustrated the importance of history-taking as a diagnostic tool. Although ultimate diagnosis required further laboratory investigations, the history indicated an overall loss of water and chronic medication use. The history of anemia and gastritis suggested that this patient's use of analgesics already had compromised her health to some degree. Finally, the case illustrated that the kidneys themselves can cause urinary frequency if they are not functioning correctly. Any kidney problem that impairs the ability of the nephron to concentrate urine results in increased urinary output.

CHAPTER 12

Chief Complaint: Decreased Visual Acuity

CASE 12-1

INITIAL PRESENTATION

Ms. B., a 24-year-old artist, presents because she "cannot see" her work. Over the past few months, she has found it increasingly difficult to see the fine details of her paintings. She is now very concerned that this problem may jeopardize her career.

1. How should care of this type of patient proceed?
2. Should the patient be referred to a specialist?

Discussion

In many cases, an internist's job is to determine which specialist is the most effective for diagnosis or treatment of a patient and to make a referral. Because no one can be an expert at everything, this is an essential function. However, determining which specialist is the most appropriate is not always easy. In addition, it is important to rule out any causes that can be handled appropriately by an internist. In this case, for example, the first instinct might be to refer this individual to an ophthalmologist for a workup. Although this may ultimately be necessary because of the expertise of an ophthalmologist in this area, there are several "internal medicine" disorders that can result in decreased visual acuity. The approach to a patient such as this is no different than the approaches analyzed throughout this book. First, the character of the symptoms must be clearly understood (i.e., what precisely does the patient mean by "worsening vision"). Also, the pattern of the symptomology can be helpful. Lastly, an understanding of any associated symptoms is particularly important in the workup of vision problems because if this symptom is the result of pathology in a different organ of the body, patients often have other complaints.

3. How will clarifying the nature of her decreased visual acuity help in differentiating a diagnosis?

Upon further inquiry, the physician discovers that the patient actually is having difficulty seeing because of double vision (diplopia). At times she is able to reduce the severity of this symptom by holding her head in a particular position. She notes no blurring, darkening, reduction in visual field, or other ophthalmologic problems. When asked about other symptoms, the patient reports that she has felt increasingly nervous lately. She has attributed this to concern about the worsening of her vision and not being able to paint. In addition, Ms. B. states that she has had several bouts of "chest palpitations." She also reports an increase in the frequency of bowel movements and a decrease in the frequency and duration of her menstrual periods over the past few months. She has no other complaints or known medical conditions, and she takes no medications.

> **Even nonspecific and disparate symptoms may, in combination, be very helpful.**

There are many problems that can result in decreased visual acuity. Diplopia implies that the eyes are not coordinating the direction of gaze. Normally, both eyes point in the same direction. However, a disturbance of conjugate gaze usually results in a complaint of double vision. This type of disturbance can result from a neurologic disorder that affects the third, fourth, or sixth cranial nerve or from a dysfunction of any of the ocular muscles.

4. Do the patient's other, less dramatic symptoms fit with her diplopia?

Of particular note is that the associated symptoms involve a very diverse group of systems, including psychologic, cardiac, gastrointestinal, and reproductive. As has been seen in many other of the cases in this book, disturbances of one system can influence other systems. Cardiac failure, for example, may result in pulmonary congestion. In this case, not one but many different systems appear to be involved, raising the suspicion of a global pathology or a single problem within a global system. An endocrine disturbance, for example, often involves many systems because of the wide-ranging and often dispersed effects of hormones. In particular, palpitations, nervousness, frequent bowel movements, and menstrual disturbances all are manifestations of a generalized hypermetabolic state that might be seen with increased thyroid hormone blood levels.

PHYSICAL EXAMINATION

The patient is an alert, young, pleasant woman who appears mildly anxious. Ms. B.'s vital signs show a regular pulse of 98 beats/min. Her blood pressure, respirations, and temperature are within normal limits. Her hair texture is unusually fine. Exophthalmos is present bilaterally with the left side greater than the right. The patient reports widening diplopia when glancing slightly upward, and there appears to be limited ocular movement on the left side, particularly when trying to look upward. The patient also exhibits difficulty with convergence. Both eyelids are slightly reddened. There is prominent lid lag bilaterally. Examination of her ears, nose, and throat is unremarkable. Her thyroid gland is enlarged bilaterally to roughly twice the normal size. It feels smooth and soft and is somewhat asymmetric. Her chest is clear to auscultation bilaterally in all fields. Her heart beat is rapid but regular without murmurs, gallops, or rubs. Examination of her abdomen is unremarkable. There is no edema or cyanosis of her extremities. Her skin is warm and moist. There is a slight, fine tremor bilaterally when the patient is asked to hold her hands in a still position. Reflexes are 2+ and equal bilaterally but exhibit a rapid return. The remainder of the physical examination is unremarkable.

5. How has this new information helped in forming a diagnosis?
6. Can a diagnosis or a determination of what abnormal physiology might be in play be made at this point?

Discussion

As is true in most of the cases encountered in internal medicine, the physical examination is mainly confirmatory. It is unusual to uncover something clinically significant yet totally unexpected during the physical examination. Most of the time, objective data are used to confirm or invalidate a working hypothesis. In this case, the physical examination confirms that this woman is suffering from thyrotoxicosis. The rapid pulse rate and fine tremor reflect the effects of thyroid hormone on the nervous and muscular systems. Although the exact mechanism is not well understood, the thyroid hormones sensitize peripheral tissues to catecholamines. Many manifestations of hyperthyroidism are similar to those seen when the adrenal medulla produces excess catecholamines. However, production of these hormones is clearly not increased in patients with an increased level of thyroid hormone. Some of these symptoms are at least partially ameliorated by β-antagonists. This is clearly not the whole story, however. The dose-response curve of epinephrine is not altered by different levels of thyroid hormone. Similarly, the exact cause of the short relaxation phase (rapid return) of the deep tendon reflexes also is unclear, but this finding is one of the hallmarks of hyperthyroidism.

The ophthalmologic abnormalities are also tell-tale signs. Lid lag occurs in all states of thyroid hormone excess and refers to the eyelid lagging behind the eyeball movement. It is detected by observing a rim of sclera between the eyelid and the limbus when the patient follows an object from a superior to an inferior gaze position. Lid lag (or the reverse, globe lag) is caused by retraction of the upper eyelid, which also may result in the bright-eyed stare of thyrotoxicosis. Lid retraction usually resolves when thyroid hormone levels are normalized, which is one reason why it is important to distinguish this finding from exophthalmos or other manifestations of Graves' disease that tend to be independent from the thyroid hormone levels. There are several causes of thyrotoxicosis, but Graves' disease (also known as diffuse thyrotoxic goiter) is the most common. It is most likely caused by autoantibodies (against the thyroid hormones) that stimulate the gland in the same manner as thyroid-stimulating hormone (TSH). The clinical complex of exophthalmos and other ocular abnormalities encountered in patients with Graves' disease is known as infiltrative ophthalmopathy, and it is usually unaffected by treatment of thyrotoxicosis. In some cases, infiltrative ophthalmopathy actually occurs in euthyroid patients. The exact pathology of this disorder is not known, but probably involves autoantibodies that attack the tissues around the eye.

Swelling of the retro-orbital fat pads and extraocular muscles is present to some degree in almost all patients with Graves' disease. Swelling of the retro-orbital fat pads causes exophthalmos, which is almost always bilateral but often worse on one side. Exophthalmometers can be used to evaluate the degree of ocular protrusion. As in this case, extraocular muscle weakness may result in diplopia by limiting the movement of one eye relative to the other. Limitations of upward gaze and convergence are the most common manifestations. The degree of infiltrative ophthalmopathy varies widely from symptoms that are barely noticeable to those that can seriously and permanently impair vision. In rare cases, the disorder may actually threaten a patient's life.

7. Are there other tests to evaluate hyperthyroid states and, if so, are they needed here?

In most clear-cut cases of Graves' disease, the serum thyroxine (T_4) level is elevated. A free T_4 is also useful to eliminate the possibility of increased levels of bound hormone (only the unbound thyroid hormones are active). Serum triiodothyronine (T_3) levels are nearly always elevated, and the TSH level is suppressed. Occasionally only the T_3 is elevated, and the T_4 is normal (often called T_3 toxicosis). If, however, the TSH is not suppressed, one should question the diagnosis of hyperthyroidism. Secondary hyperthyroidism from a TSH-secreting tumor is an extremely rare condition in which the TSH, T_4, and T_3 levels are elevated. A radioactive iodine uptake (RAIU) study is useful to distinguish between true hyperthyroidism, as in Graves' disease, and thyroiditis.

In patients with thyroiditis, the gland may release large amounts of T_4 into the circulation, causing a temporary (perhaps 4–6 week) hyperthyroidism. During the hyperactive phase of thyroiditis, the RAIU will be low, an apparent paradox. The explanation is that thyroiditis consists of periods of making thyroid hormone and storing it and then releasing hormone and not making it. In true hyperthyroidism, elevated blood levels of thyroid hormone are accompanied by increased hormone production, and this is reflected in a high RAIU. In addition, a RAIU study with a scan may be helpful if a goiter is asymmetrical to rule out toxic adenomas or trophoblastic tumors. In this case, however, RAIU would not be necessary or recommended because the patient has signs and symptoms of Graves' disease. Infiltrative ophthalmology with exophthalmos is not part of thyroiditis.

Laboratory evaluation for thyrotoxicosis is most valuable in cases in which the symptoms are mild or the diagnosis is in question. The symptoms of hyperthyroidism vary greatly in terms of both number and severity. As a result, diagnostic approaches also may vary. In this case, the clear indications of infiltrative ophthalmopathy make a diagnosis of Graves' disease virtually certain even before laboratory testing. However, in other patients, diseases such as anxiety disorders or pheochromocytoma also may be suspected and, in those cases, thyroid testing is essential to differentiate the conditions.

8. How should Ms. B. be treated?

The treatment of hyperthyroidism is as variable as the symptomology and underlying causes. Thyroidectomy, ablation with radioactive iodine (^{131}I), and iodine uptake–blocking drug therapy all are effective in different circumstances. Propylthiouracil and methimazole inhibit the incorporation of iodine into tyrosine and therefore retard the production of thyroid hormone. In addition, methimazole may actually decrease levels of antimicrosomal and anti-TSH antibodies, which are thought to be responsible for thyroid stimulation in patients with Graves' disease. One advantage to drug therapy is that after 6–18 months, treatment often can be discontinued without thyroid replacement. However, patients should be monitored closely because many Graves' disease patients, even treated with "nonpermanent" antithyroid drugs, eventually become hypothyroid. Often, hypothyroidism occurs years after the initial patient presentation. The disadvantages of drug therapy are possible side effects, including the rare but very serious bone marrow depression, recurrence of disease, and the need for continuous monitoring. Beta-blockers may be helpful to ameliorate some symptoms immediately prior to achieving a euthyroid state, which may not occur for weeks or months.

Surgery is another therapeutic approach to this type of patient. Subtotal thyroidectomy is theoretically more permanent than treatment with antithyroid agents. However, it does have some disadvantages. The patient should be treated preoperatively for at least 2 weeks with beta-blockers and antithyroid drugs to reduce the risk of thyroid storm, which is a condition of severe thyrotoxicosis that can be life-threatening and may be induced by anesthesia or surgery. The most common adverse event following surgery is permanent hypothyroidism. Recurrence of thyrotoxicosis occurs in a smaller percentage of cases. In addition to problems that may occur with any surgical patient (e.g., anesthetic events, bleeding, infection), other adverse events may arise that are unique to thyroid surgery due to its anatomic position in the neck. These include recurrent laryngeal nerve damage and hypoparathyroidism.

Treatment with ^{131}I is yet another therapeutic possibility. The thyroid gland is the only tissue in the body that actively takes up iodine. As a result, the thyroid gland can be ablated with ^{131}I without an increased risk of cancer in the thyroid or other organs. There are three possible side effects of ^{131}I ablation. The first is the risk of hypothyroidism, which is a concern with all modalities of treatment. The second is an unproved possibility of genetic damage to gametes. To date, there is no convincing evidence of any direct relationship between ^{131}I ablation and genetic damage. However, the amount of radiation that is necessary to disrupt genetic coding has never been established. For this reason, ^{131}I therapy should not be used in pregnant women. The third potential problem with ^{131}I ablation has been reported only recently and is not universally accepted. In these studies, patients treated with ^{131}I had worsening of existing ophthalmopathy compared to those treated with blocking drugs. [131]I therapy is the treatment of choice for individuals who have had recurrence of hyperthyroidism after surgery.

Unfortunately, treatment of infiltrative ophthalmopathy may be extremely difficult. As discussed earlier, eye involvement occurs independently from the thyroid hormone levels and does not resolve with antithyroid treatment. In addition, the course of the disease is quite variable, and the effectiveness of treatment is debatable. Treatment of mild symptoms is generally palliative until symptoms remit. Hydrating eye drops, for example, often may provide relief of eye irritation. For more severe cases, glucocorticoids and external radiation therapy may be effective. Occasionally, surgical decompression of the orbit is necessary. When the exophthalmos is advanced, eye drops and nocturnal eye patches may be critical to prevent corneal drying and permanent damage.

ASSESSMENT

Ms. B. is diagnosed with **Graves' disease with ophthalmopathy.** Her treatment plan includes T_4, T_3, and TSH. She should then begin beta-blocker therapy in the form of 10 mg propranolol orally three times a day. If the laboratory tests indicate significant hyperthyroidism, she should begin 15 mg methimazole orally each morning until it is determined what therapeutic modality is preferred for long-term care. The patient should be referred to an ophthalmologist to assess the degree of ophthalmopathy and followed for possible intervention.

CASE 12-2

INITIAL PRESENTATION

A 22-year-old man complains of an episode of visual problems associated with a headache. The symptoms started this morning with "difficulty seeing," which the patient describes as "stars, sparks, and shapes moving all around." The symptoms came on slowly and have worsened progressively until seeing any fine detail was impossible. Within 1 hour, the visual symptoms resolved spontaneously. After roughly 15 minutes, the patient experienced a severe, right-sided, throbbing headache, which was exacerbated by light and physical activity. The patient is now symptom free but presents to the internal medicine clinic because he is worried about what happened. The patient has no significant medical history. The patient denies alcohol or drug use.

PHYSICAL EXAMINATION

The young man appears anxious but is otherwise well nourished and healthy. Vision tests show 20/20 acuity bilaterally. Visual fields are full by confrontation. Extraocular movements are intact. Funduscopic examination shows clear sharp disks without evidence of retinal problems. The corneas and sclera are clear. The neurologic examination is completely within normal limits. The remainder of the physical examination is unremarkable. The patient is asymptomatic at the time of the examination.

ASSESSMENT

There are a few interesting aspects of this case that give some indication of a possible diagnosis. In this case, there are few concerns regarding risk factors. A young man without a history of medical illness is not at known increased risk of serious illness. In addition, the physical examination is unremarkable, suggesting that the disorder either is intermittent or not globally pernicious enough to cause physical abnormalities. In this case, the pattern of presentation and associated symptoms are perhaps the most helpful. A throbbing headache often suggests vascular involvement. As mentioned in other chapters of this book, unilateral headache implies a somewhat localized event. It is worth noting that the pattern of visual disturbance is "positive." In other words, the visual defects do not consist of any absences in the visual field, but instead are "additions" (i.e., stars, sparks, shapes) to the normal pattern of sight. It is possible that the patient is having psychotic hallucinations, but with no history of psychiatric disease or drug use, this diagnosis is less likely. "Negative" visual dysfunction can be a clue to nerve impingement or retinal problems such as detachment or ischemia.

The chronologic pattern also is a clue. Visual disturbances followed by a throbbing headache are highly suspicious of a **migraine.** Migraine headache is discussed elsewhere in this book (see Chapter 6), but it is worth noting that although many patients suffer from chronic migraines, patients occasionally present with an initial episode at almost any time in life. If this is indeed a migraine, this patient may or may not have any future episodes. As a result, patient education is helpful. An explanation of the sequence in a migraine episode may help reassure the patient. The spasm of arteries serving the occipital lobe of the brain usually is unilateral, and the resultant relative ischemia causes the visual disturbance. When the arterial spasms resolve, the vision clears, but the relaxation of the arteries is associated with a unilateral throbbing headache. The events, although disturbing and painful, rarely have any sequelae. Given the lack of other findings in this case and the "textbook" presentation, further investigation of a migraine headache probably is not warranted unless the patient experiences future problems, especially visual deterioration or neurologic disturbances. Occasionally, patients experience painless migraines in which the visual disturbances are not followed by headache. This is sometimes confusing to the diagnostician but is otherwise no different from the usual migraine.

This patient should be educated; the physician should explain the disorder and address any pattern of environmental triggers or stress, if feasible. If the migraines recur, a program of prevention with medication such as beta-blockers may be necessary.

CASE 12-3

INITIAL PRESENTATION

A 44-year-old man presents with difficulty seeing. The patient is a city bus driver and over the past 6 months has noticed increasing difficulty seeing when changing lanes and turning. He states that the other day he almost pulled out in front of an oncoming vehicle when trying to turn left onto a busy street. He denies blurred vision or decreased visual acuity when looking directly at an object. However, he notes that he often has difficulty locating objects in the periphery. The patient also complains of dull headaches over the same time period in the midfrontal region, which seem to be increasing in intensity. The patient reveals that he is recently divorced from his wife. He states that part of his marital problem was that he has not had any interest in sexual activity for more than 1 year. In addition, he has noticed an increasing lack of energy over the past year, but has attributed this to his marital difficulties. He also has noticed some progressively worsening cold intolerance.

PHYSICAL EXAMINATION

The patient's vital signs are: temperature, 97°F; respirations, 18 breaths/min; blood pressure, 128/88 mm Hg (supine) and 110/72 mm Hg standing; and pulse, 76 beats/min supine and 106 beats/min standing, with subjective lightheadedness. The patient appears somewhat lethargic but is otherwise in no apparent distress. Examination of his head, ears, nose, and throat is unremarkable. Examination of his eyes reveals intact extraocular movements; however, visual fields are decreased in the upper lateral areas by confrontation. The retinas appear normal with sharp disks. His neck is supple with no thyromegaly or lymphadenopathy. A chest examination reveals notable gynecomastia, but no galactorrhea. His lungs are clear to percussion and auscultation. A cardiac examination indicates a normal first (S_1) and second (S_2) heart sound with no murmurs. An abdominal examination is unremarkable. Examination of his genitals reveals a normal male escutcheon. His penis and testes appear normal. There is no cyanosis or edema in the extremities. His reflexes are all 2+ but exhibit a delayed return. The remainder of the physical examination is unremarkable.

ASSESSMENT

There are several aspects of this case that help in reaching a preliminary diagnosis. First, as in the other cases in this chapter, the precise visual problem is important. The history and physical examination suggest that this patient has a temporal hemianopsia, particularly superiorly. In other words, he has at least partial blindness bilaterally to peripheral vision. This suggests a problem in or around the optic chiasm. Light from the peripheral field hits the medial portion of the retina. This signal is then carried via the optic nerve to the optic chiasm, where the nerve pathways cross before being carried to the lateral geniculate bodies. As a result, a lesion in the area of the optic chiasm can result in an inability to perceive objects in the temporal or peripheral region of vision.

In addition to the type of visual disturbance, the pattern of disease onset is helpful in determining the pathologic process involved. This patient's symptoms began months ago and have progressively gotten worse. A chronic pathology makes a neoplastic or degenerative process more likely than an infectious, vascular, or traumatic process.

The third aspect of this case that is particularly helpful is similar to that noted in the previous case; that is, a variety of systems seem to be affected. The temporal hemianopsia and midfrontal headache are consistent with an optic chiasm problem. Decreased energy, dry skin, and slow-returning reflexes indicate possible hypothyroidism. Decreased libido and gynecomastia imply a dysfunction of sex hormones. Lastly, orthostatic hypotension suggests a neurologic, vascular contractility, or hypovolemic problem, possibly related to a dysfunction of the renin-angiotensin-aldosterone system. As in the previous case, it is certainly possible for a single patient to have multiple problems. However, it is less likely for several different problems to begin simultaneously unless there is a common or overlapping pathology. When many different systems seem to be involved, it is often productive to examine the possibility of a global pathology, such as an autoimmune problem or dysfunction of a system that can have global effects, such as an endocrine disorder.

In this case, there appears to be clear indication of several endocrine imbalances, and an endocrine etiology is therefore likely.

The next step is to look at the pattern of the various endocrine imbalances. All of the symptoms, with the exception of gynecomastia, are consistent with hypofunctioning endocrine glands. An across-the-board decrease in peripheral hormones should raise suspicion of a hypopituitary state. Gynecomastia, on the other hand, suggests an increase in either prolactin or estrogen (at least relative to testosterone). When taken together, the most likely diagnosis is a **prolactin-secreting pituitary adenoma.** This is a space-occupying lesion that puts pressure on the optic chiasm, resulting in bilateral temporal blindness. Pituitary cells producing TSH, luteinizing hormone (LH), follicle-stimulating hormone (FSH), and adrenocorticotropic hormone (ACTH) are crowded by the expanding adenoma, resulting in decreased production of these hormones. Measuring hormone levels and magnetic resonance imaging of the pituitary gland would be the next steps toward diagnosis. A proper visual field study should also be performed to document the degree of visual impairment. Eventually, treatment with surgery, radiation, or dopamine agonists along with hormone replacement therapy will be necessary. If the prolactin level is quite high, the testosterone is suppressed and may increase concomitant with lowering the prolactin level. Sometimes this results in improvement of sexual function and gynecomastia without testosterone supplementation.

CASE 12-4

INITIAL PRESENTATION

A 48-year-old man with type 2 diabetes mellitus (type 2 DM) complains of "having trouble seeing." The patient states that he has noticed frequent episodes of blurred vision over the past 2–3 weeks. The symptoms wax and wane throughout the day, but some degree of blurring is almost always present. The patient has worn glasses all of his adult life. He sees an ophthalmologist annually, and he finds this new difficulty strange because his physician told him that his prescription did not need changing at his last visit 2 months ago. According to the patient's chart, the ophthalmologist found no signs of retinopathy during a dilated ophthalmologic examination. The patient had been on sulfonylurea medications to treat his type 2 DM until last month, when he was converted to insulin therapy to control his sugar levels better.

PHYSICAL EXAMINATION

A physical examination is completely unremarkable, including a careful funduscopic evaluation.

ASSESSMENT

Diabetes (particularly type 1 DM) is the leading cause of adult blindness in the United States. As a result, retinopathy is always a concern. Fortunately, this patient has been seeing an ophthalmologist regularly. A dilated ophthalmologic examination by a specialist is far more sensitive than an in-office examination of the fundi. For this reason, it is recommended that all diabetics see an ophthalmologist on an annual basis. Because the most recent examination was normal in this case, retinopathy is most unlikely. Again, the pattern of the symptomology is important. This problem had a relatively acute onset, suggesting an acute etiology. Therefore, it is more likely that the **recent change in this individual's diabetes management is affecting his vision.** Changes in blood sugar levels can acutely affect vision because of the osmotic properties of glucose. In the eye, elevated levels of glucose draw water into the aqueous and vitreous humors, altering the distance to the retina. As a result, the focal point is moved, and vision is blurred. As this patient's sugar level became increasingly high, his vision probably changed very gradually so that he did not notice it. His glasses most likely were made to correct for the influence of the elevated sugar in addition to his primary lens problem. However, he was recently placed on insulin, which could have acutely lowered his sugar levels. This would have relatively quickly changed the osmotic pressures in his eyes, altered the fluid in the humors, and changed his focal point. As a result, his current eyeglass prescription does not correct for the current focal point, and his vision is blurred. Because appropriate glucose control may be crucial for delaying the onset of retinopathy, the priority here is control of his diabetes. Once his blood sugar levels are stabilized in an appropriate range for 4–6 weeks, the patient can see his ophthalmologist, and a new prescription for glasses should resolve his visual problems.

CASE 12-5

INITIAL PRESENTATION

A 78-year-old man presents complaining of difficulty reading. The patient's peripheral vision is "fine," but he has been noticing increasing difficulty seeing objects in the center of his visual field. The actual description of the visual impairment is difficult for the patient to describe. He states that objects in the center of his visual field, "just do not seem to be there" (central scotoma). The problem began insidiously and has been increasingly noticeable over the past year. The patient has no other remarkable medical history.

PHYSICAL EXAMINATION

The patient is well nourished and in no apparent distress. He tilts his head and eyes to the left side when looking at objects. Acuity is 20/400 bilaterally. His extraocular movements are intact. Peripheral visual fields are full by confrontation. Funduscopic examination reveals dark mottling around the macula bilaterally. The remainder of the physical examination is unremarkable.

ASSESSMENT

There are two primary distinctions in this case. The first is the ever-present concern of risk factors. The only risk factor here is the patient's age. However, this is a risk factor that should not be overlooked. Visual changes in the elderly are a major focus of many internal medicine practices. The elderly are at risk for a variety of vision problems such as cataracts, presbyopia, macular degeneration, and glaucoma. In addition, the elderly are at higher risk from visual complications of chronic illnesses, such as diabetes, simply because the elderly have had such diseases for longer periods of time.

The second distinction in this case (as seen elsewhere in this chapter) is the pattern of the visual impairment. Loss of central vision indicates a dysfunction of the central portion of the retina. This area, known as the macula, has a higher concentration of cones and is therefore normally needed for clear color vision of fine details. Because this patient's peripheral vision is intact, we may infer that the outer portion of the retinas is spared. This presentation is typical of **macular degeneration.** The etiology of this disorder is unclear, and unfortunately, treatment usually is ineffective. Management consists of preventing other ocular damage and making the most out of the peripheral vision that is available. The patient should be referred to an ophthalmologist for confirmation of the diagnosis.

SUMMARY

There are a variety of visual complaints that may be encountered by an internist. The approach to a visually impaired patient should not be dramatically different from the approach to any other internal medicine patient. Of primary importance is the determination of exactly what the patient is describing. Scotomas, hallucinations, diplopia, and blurred vision all can have markedly different etiologies, and diagnosis is impossible without a clear understanding of the visual problem. In addition, a risk factor assessment coupled with the pattern of presentation can be a powerful tool in making a correct diagnosis. Sudden onset of visual impairment in a young person following a racquetball injury raises concerns about retinal detachment, but slowly progressing decreased visual acuity in an elderly patient with diabetes is much more likely to be a degenerative process such as diabetic retinopathy. After an initial history and physical examination, an internist must then decide how to proceed. In some cases, an "internal medicine" etiology can be ruled in, and care can be initiated. In other cases, however, specialized ophthalmologic care is required, and the internist must function in a triage capacity. Visual symptoms often can be clues to global problems, but at some point, an ophthalmologist must be involved to ensure that the patient's eyesight is not jeopardized.

CHAPTER 13

Chief Complaint: Nausea and Vomiting

CASE 13-1

INITIAL PRESENTATION

Mr. D., a 43-year-old bartender, comes into an internal medicine clinic with a chief complaint of nausea and vomiting of 2 weeks duration. The patient states that he has noticed increasing fatigue over the last month. Roughly 3 weeks ago he began to notice muscle and joint aches, which he attributed to "the flu." Within the last 2 weeks, the patient has noticed the gradual onset of nausea, loss of appetite, and abdominal pain. The nausea does not seem to be affected by food intake. The patient has vomited three or four times over the past week and tells you of some slight chills. He denies vomiting blood or coffee-grounds material. He states that his stools have been loose but that he has not had frank diarrhea. He has no personal or family history of gallstones. Further questioning reveals that the patient has noticed that his urine has been darker than usual lately. He denies any other changes in urinary habits.

> There is a gradual onset of symptoms.

1. What systems can be involved in the presentation of nausea and vomiting?
2. How has the information related by the patient helped you?

Discussion

Vomiting is the expulsion of gastric contents (as well as duodenal material in certain circumstances) through the oral cavity. It is a reflex action controlled in the medulla. Both chemical and mechanical stimulation of the vomiting centers can cause emesis. Nausea and vomiting often occur simultaneously. Although the occurrence of these symptoms is often the result of an infection of the gastrointestinal (GI) tract, nausea and vomiting can also occur from disturbances of the GI, psychiatric, cardiac, endocrine/metabolic, genitourinary, and central nervous (CNS) systems. Fortunately, the symptomology is frequently straightforward, and an appropriate history and physical are often all that are needed for the initial diagnosis.

While CNS disorders (such as stroke) may cause nausea and vomiting, other CNS manifestations usually prevail and thus the diagnosis is obvious. Anxiety disorders may also present with nausea, but similarly, other manifestations clarify the diagnosis. Barring these exceptions, most cases of nausea and vomiting involve the GI tract either primarily or secondarily. This is supported in this case by the history of abdominal pain. The presence of fever should always raise suspicion of some type of infection or inflammation. It is also worth noting that this patient's problems worsened gradually, suggesting a chronic, insidious process. The fact that the nausea does not worsen with food intake may indicate that the "true" GI tract may be spared. Typically, disturbances in the esophagus, stomach, and small or large intestine result in symptoms that are changed in one way or another with differing food intake. However, this is a very soft symptom. The presence of arthralgias and myalgias is potentially helpful, but since these symptoms are very common manifestations of any infection, the significance must be regarded with caution. Many times, these symptoms signify a systemic immune reaction. The presence of dark urine may be quite helpful. Generally this finding indicates the presence of one of four things in the urine: relative increase in solute (from dehydration), blood, metabolite or toxin, or bilirubin. Without evidence of dehydration, kidney problems, or exogenous substance, dark urine may signify hepatic dysfunction.

3. After considering this possibility and carefully examining this patient's eyes, which reveal slightly yellow sclera, what would you do next?

At this point, the finding of icteric sclera makes a hepatic etiology even more likely. If hepatitis is suspected, the history can be directed to ascertain the source of infection. In this case, a risk factor assessment would be very important. Mr. D. does not drink alcohol, does not take any medications regularly including over-the-counter pain relievers such as acetaminophen, and has no history of exposure to chemical toxins such as industrial solvents. The patient tells you that he has not changed his dietary habits at all. He has not traveled recently and has not been in any unsanitary conditions. Also, no one with whom he has

> There is no evidence of alcoholic or toxic hepatitis.

been in contact is ill. He likes to pre-
pare his own meals and is careful to
wash and cook everything thoroughly.
Mr. D. states that he has no history of
operations, has never had a blood
transfusion, and has never used intravenous (IV) drugs. Further questioning
reveals that Mr. D. is homosexual. He

> There is no evi-
> dence of fecal-
> oral infection or
> hepatitis A
> (HAV) or E
> (HEV).

has engaged in sexual activity with numerous men throughout the
course of his adult life. He has not had any long-term relationships
and does not regularly use condoms.

Obviously, the patient's high-risk be-
havior raises some definite concerns. A
risk factor assessment not only provides key clues to the diagnosis but can
also help with long-term care of patients. Different disease entities affect
different population groups due to age,
race, genetics, geographic location,
living-working environment, and life-
style. Homosexual men who do not

> Hepatitis C
> (HCV) is a major
> cause of post-
> transfusion hep-
> atitis. The virus
> can also be
> spread via other
> types of blood or
> sexual contact.

practice protected sex are at higher risk for many diseases including
HBV and HCV, gonorrhea, *Shigella*,
Campylobacter, *Entamoeba*, *Giardia*, and
human immunodeficiency virus (HIV).
In addition to treatment for his current
illness, this patient may need testing
for the other diseases and should be educated about the dangers he poses to
himself and others.

> Unprotected sex-
> ual activity is a
> major risk factor
> for hepatitis B
> (HBV) and to a
> lesser extent
> HCV.

PHYSICAL EXAMINATION

The patient is a somewhat thin man who appears his stated age and
seems to be in mild distress. His temperature is 101°F.; blood pressure,
pulse, and respirations are within normal limits. The eyes are remarkable for icteric sclera. The throat is clear without erythema or exudate.
The remainder of the head, ears, eyes, nose, and throat (HEENT) examination is unremarkable. His neck is supple without thyromegaly or
adenopathy. No carotid bruits are heard. Close examination shows
slight jaundice but no rashes or lesions. His lungs are clear, and his
heart examination is unremarkable. Abdominal examination reveals
normal bowel sounds. The liver is enlarged to 16 cm at the midclavicu-
lar line and is tender. There is also some diffuse tenderness to palpation throughout the abdomen. Murphy's sign is negative. No masses
or splenomegaly were noted. No abdominal bruits are heard. Rectal

examination is normal, and the stool is a normal brown color and guaiac negative. Extremities show no clubbing, cyanosis, or edema. The neurological examination is unremarkable.

> 4. How has the information from the physical examination helped you?

Discussion

The physical examination findings help confirm the hypothesis of hepatitis. The slightly elevated temperature is consistent with the patient's complaint of chills. The icteric sclera and jaundice support a hepatic etiology. Occasionally, gallstones obstruct the common bile duct and cause jaundice and right upper quadrant pain. However, this usually results in light-colored stools and a positive Murphy's sign (presence of sharp pain felt on deep inspiration with palpation under the right anterior rib cage). In addition, this patient has no history of gallbladder disease. The diagnosis of hepatitis is strongly supported by the findings of a tender, enlarged liver. The next step is to determine what kind of hepatitis this patient has. Risk factors suggest that HBV would be most likely; however, it would be reasonable at this point to assess the degree of liver damage and to test for other diseases for which the patient may be at high risk such as HCV and HIV.

LABORATORY TESTS

Laboratory tests results are listed below.

Laboratory Tests	Patient	Normal Values
Aspartate transaminase (AST)	500 IU/L	10–30 IU/L
Alanine transaminase (ALT)	530 IU/L	8–20 IU/L
γ-Glutamyltransferase (GGT)	35 IU/L	9–50 IU/L
Alkaline phosphatase	195 IU/L	53–128 IU/L
Total bilirubin	3.0 mg/dL	0.2–1.0 mg/dL
Direct bilirubin	2.8 mg/dL	Less than 0.2 mg/dL
HAV IgG and IgM	Negative	Negative
Hepatitis B surface antigen (HBsAg)	Positive	Negative
Hepatitis B e antigen (HBeAg)	Positive	Negative
Hepatitis B core antibody (Anti-HBc)	Positive	Negative
Hepatitis B e antibody (Anti-HBe)	Negative	Negative
Hepatitis B surface antibody (Anti-HBs)	Negative	Negative
Delta hepatitis (HDV) IgM and IgG	Negative	Negative
Anti-HCV	Negative	Negative
HCV RNA	Negative	Negative
HIV	Negative	Negative
Albumin	3.5 g/dL	3.5–5.0 g/dL
White blood cells (WBCs) [increased neutrophils]	11,000/mm³	4500–11,000/mm³
Urinalysis shows 2+ bilirubin but is otherwise normal.		

5. How would you interpret these laboratory findings?

Discussion

To understand the significance of each of these tests, we will analyze them one at a time. AST and ALT are enzymes that are prevalent in liver cells. When these cells are damaged, these enzymes spill into the serum. As a result, elevated levels are a nonspecific indication of acute hepatocellular damage. There is some variability of the ratio. AST tends to be a more sensitive indicator of alcoholic damage, while ALT is often more elevated in biliary obstructive disorders. Alkaline phosphatase and GGT are also enzymes that are found in high quantities in hepatocytes. While any damage to liver cells can cause an increase in the serum levels of these factors, biliary obstructive disorders, as with gallstones in the common bile duct, cause especially high levels. The relatively small increases in this case indicate that biliary obstruction or stasis is not a major factor thus far in the progression of this patient's disease. This fact is also supported by the absence of pale-colored stools, since bilirubin and urobilinogen (a bacterial metabolite of bilirubin) give stool its color.

The total and direct bilirubin findings are consistent with what we know already, and help confirm the diagnosis of acute hepatitis. Direct bilirubin refers to the fraction of the total amount of bilirubin that is conjugated with glucuronic acid. Bilirubin by itself is not soluble in aqueous solutions. When red blood cells (RBCs) are broken down in the spleen, bilirubin is bound to albumin in the serum to be transported to the liver. In the liver, bilirubin is conjugated with glucuronic acid so that it can be excreted in the bile. Since conjugation is necessary for solubility, the presence of bilirubin in the urine indicates that conjugation is occurring. In other words, we know from the history of dark urine and the finding of bilirubin in the urine that conjugation is not the problem. This is consistent with the diagnosis of hepatitis, since the major dysfunction in this disorder is an inability to transport conjugated bilirubin into the bile. In severe cases, the transport may be inhibited to the extent that stools will appear pale. In other disorders such as massive hemolysis of RBCs or newborn jaundice, the primary problem is an elevation of unconjugated hemoglobin. As a result, patients with these disorders do not have histories of dark urine.

The negative HAV and HDV antibody titers confirm that this patient has not contracted HAV or HDV. Similarly, the absence of HCV antibodies and RNA help rule out chronic and acute infection from this virus. HDV is thought to be associated with increased virulence of HBV when co-infection occurs.

The HBsAg and HbeAg are positive, indicating active infection. The HBcAg is also present but is rendered undetectable by the core antibody, which is nonprotective and generally occurs early in the course of the disease. Core antibody may remain elevated for many years following the initial infection, making this an excellent marker for previous exposure. Alternatively, antibodies against the envelope and the surface of the virus are protective. Their presence usually indicates the end of the active phase. Therefore, it is not surprising that these titers are negative early in the disease course. Roughly 10% of individuals with HBV will develop chronic active hepatitis. In such individuals, HbsAg remains in the serum and anti-HBc never appears.

As always, elevations in the WBC count indicate infection or inflammation. In most cases of acute hepatitis, the WBC count is in the upper limits of normal or is mildly elevated. Low-normal values in the presence of disease should raise suspicion of a weakened immune response.

Among its many other functions, the liver produces a great many proteins for use in other areas of the body. Therefore, liver damage can decrease the serum levels of such proteins as albumin. You may recall that patients with cirrhosis of the liver often develop ascites, indicating that the serum protein levels are so low that the osmotic pressure within the vasculature is no longer high enough to keep fluid from leaking into the peritoneal cavity.

ASSESSMENT

As with all viral infections the treatment of HBV is largely supportive. A high-calorie diet may be helpful. Corticosteroid therapy should be avoided because it may increase the severity of chronic disease. Clearly, the most important medical intervention for this patient's long-term survival would be preventive education. An explanation of the cause of Mr. D.'s infection is vital to prevent other sexually transmitted diseases (STDs) and to prevent the spread of the disease to others. Extensive education regarding his risks of contracting additional infections and life-style changes to prevent the spread of **HBV** from him to others are necessary.

CASE 13-2

INITIAL PRESENTATION

A 24-year-old woman presents to an urgent care clinic with a chief complaint of nausea and vomiting beginning this morning.

The patient felt fine for most of the previous day but went to bed early because she was tired. She woke up with fever, chills, abdominal pain, nausea, and diarrhea, and since then, she has vomited several times. She noted no blood or coffee-grounds material in her vomit. She denies any recent travel, medications, or change in diet. The patient believes that she is suffering from "food poisoning" from chicken she had last night in a restaurant. She knows of no other patrons of the establishment becoming ill. The patient is not sexually active.

PHYSICAL EXAMINATION

Temperature is 100.4°F. Her skin is negative for tenting. Mucous membranes are moist. Bowel sounds are present, and the abdomen is soft and slightly tender to palpation diffusely. No masses or organomegaly are noted. Stool is guaiac negative. The remainder of the physical examination is unremarkable.

ASSESSMENT

It is often said that medicine is not an exact science. In fact, it probably is an exact science, but individual variation and our lack of knowledge make it appear imprecise. As a result, physicians almost never make diagnostic or therapeutic decisions with complete certainty. The most important question is: What should I do now that will result in the highest probability of achieving the desired results? In answering this question, due consideration must be given to the cost as well as the risk and discomfort to the patient of any diagnostic or therapeutic choice you make. (If doctoring were easy, everyone would be doing it.) Of all the complaints evaluated by internists, those related to the gastrointestinal (GI) tract are second in frequency only to those attributed to the respiratory system. This is a "typical" GI case, and the exact etiology is unclear at this point. Many GI infections are spread through food intake. Often, a toxin produced by bacteria is the cause, regardless of whether there are any live bacteria present. Generally, in gastroenteritis as a result of food-borne toxins, there is a relatively short (less than 6 hours) time from ingestion to illness, and vomiting is the most common symptom. Alternatively, bacterial infections take longer to manifest and usually present with diarrhea. Patients often use the term "food poisoning" to describe any kind of gastroenteritis. Clinically, however, the term is usually reserved for situations in which a definitive etiology can be established. Most of these cases involve potentially serious illnesses which must be thoroughly investigated for the health of the public. In actuality, the patient's use of the term food poisoning is usually quite correct. Mild GI symptoms acquired via food intake are extremely common, and all cases could aptly be termed "food poisoning." Fortunately, most cases are relatively benign and self-limiting, which brings us back to the question: What do we do now? This patient has acute symptoms, suggesting infection or intoxication. Many times, patients focus on their last meal (chicken dinner last night), but as a result of the variability of the incubation period, this belief may not be justified. Without signs of dehydration, bleeding, or more serious infection, it is not necessary or possible to track down the origin of the disorder. Similarly, these patients do not usually require any substantial medical intervention. Exceptions include cases of the elderly or individuals with underlying medical conditions that could predispose to serious complications. In this case, the patient is an otherwise healthy young woman without signs of dehydration and is most likely suffering from a **nonspecific, viral gastroenteritis** or mildly toxic food poisoning. A conservative approach would therefore be reasonable. Oral fluids initially (if tolerated) and antinausea medications later are usually all that are necessary. However, if symptoms should worsen or if the patient is unable to maintain adequate hydration, further steps may be necessary.

The patient is instructed to drink lots of fluids; rest; and call if symptoms worsen, hematemesis occurs, or hydration cannot be maintained. Antiemetics should be avoided during the first 24 hours since vomiting is useful in ridding the stomach of toxins.

CASE 13-3

INITIAL PRESENTATION

A 45-year-old Hispanic woman presents to the internal medicine clinic with a chief complaint of nausea, vomiting, and severe abdominal pain of 2 days duration. The nausea has been waxing and waning but is nearly always present. She has vomited three times in the last 2 days. The abdominal pain occurs episodically, usually beginning abruptly and gradually diminishing over 30 minutes to an hour. The pain is located in the right upper quadrant and occasionally radiates to the back and right shoulder. The patient has also noted some chills, which have been relieved with aspirin. She also reports slightly darker colored urine. The patient has no other medical problems and takes no medications other than aspirin for chills. The last aspirin she took was 2 hours ago. She had a tubal ligation 15 years ago. She has no history of travel, dietary changes, or other known risk factors.

PHYSICAL EXAMINATION

The patient is a mildly obese woman in obvious distress from abdominal pain and nausea. Her temperature is 99°F. The sclera are not icteric. The abdomen is diffusely tender with severe pain on deep palpation of the right upper quadrant. Guarding and rebound tenderness are also present in this region. There is also severe pain with deep inspiration during right subcostal palpation (Murphy's sign).

LABORATORY TESTS

Laboratory tests results are given in the table below.

Laboratory Tests	Patient	Normal Values
AST	75 IU/L	10–30 IU/L
ALT	104 IU/L	8–20 IU/L
GGT	30 IU/L	9–50 IU/L
Alkaline phosphatase	276 IU/L	42–98 IU/L
Total bilirubin	1.4 mg/dL	0.2–1.0 mg/dL
Direct bilirubin	1.2 mg/dL	Less than 0.2 mg/dL
WBCs	12,000	4500–11,000
Urinalysis	1+ bilirubin	none

ASSESSMENT

We have discussed elsewhere the importance of localizing abdominal pain. In this case, pain in the right upper quadrant, especially radiating to the back or shoulder, is strongly suggestive of an hepatic or gallbladder problem. A positive Murphy's sign supports gallbladder irritation. Inflammation of the gallbladder results in sharp pain with palpation and deep inspiration because contraction of the diaphragm pushes the gallbladder down against the examiner's hand. In addition, the sudden onset of severe pain raises suspicion that an obstructive pathology may be responsible. Note that although the serum bilirubin is elevated, the sclera are not icteric. The total serum bilirubin usually must be above 2.5 mg/dL before noticeable scleral icterus occurs. In Case 13-1, we discussed that bilirubin in the urine was indicative of conjugation and subsequent failure of excretion. We also noted that alkaline phosphatase is more sensitive than other liver enzymes to obstructive disorders. All of these findings together implicate **acute cholecystitis** as the cause of this woman's problems. Cholecystitis is more common in certain ethnic groups, including Hispanics.

Acute cholecystitis is almost always caused by obstruction of either the cystic duct or common bile duct (or both) by gallstones (cholelithiasis). Gallstones can generally be divided into two categories: pigment stones and cholesterol stones. The pathogenesis of pigment stones is poorly understood. They are composed of bile pigments and calcium, so they are usually radiopaque. Brown pigment stones are more common in Asians. Black pigment stones are more frequent in patients with cirrhosis and hemolytic anemia. The most common type of gallstone in industrialized areas of the world is composed of cholesterol and is not usually visible on a plain x-ray.

Because of the relative prevalence of cholesterol stones, plain abdominal x-rays are not sensitive enough for use as an initial diagnostic tool when cholecystitis is suspected. Instead, an ultrasound scan is the preferred first step. This study is noninvasive and fairly sensitive in determining the presence of gallstones and other potential causes of right upper quadrant pain. If ultrasound reveals no stones and no other abnormalities, cholescintigraphy is usually definitive in ruling in or out the suspected diagnosis. Intravenous hepatoiminodiacetic acid (HIDA) is a radioactive marker that is selectively taken up by hepatocytes and excreted into the bile. In patients without cholecystitis, the gallbladder will be illuminated after injection. In patients with cholecystitis, because of swelling or other types of blockage of the common or cystic ducts, the dye cannot be excreted into the bile or taken into the gallbladder to allow visualization.

Therapy is both medical and surgical. Most physicians agree that the patient should first be stabilized medically, and then undergo surgery for removal of the gallbladder. Medical measures may involve pain control, pharmacologic intervention for nausea and vomiting, intravenous (IV) therapy for hydration and electrolyte balance, and antibiotic treatment for individuals with fever and an elevated WBC count. Unusual causes of acute cholecystitis include infection and trauma.

Untreated acute cholecystitis has a variable course. Sepsis, with or without perforation, may occur. Infection with gas-forming bacteria such as *Clostridium* can be especially devastating. In addition, patients are at risk for the formation of fistulas connecting to the small intestine. Yet another complication is gallstone ileus, where a portion of the bowel develops a functional blockage because of irritation from the inflamed gallbladder. Along with reducing complications, laparoscopic cholecystectomy avoids chronic inflammation, which may result in permanent damage to the bile ducts necessitating the need for open cholecystectomy. The patient must be stabilized with fluids and pain medications. A surgical consultation should be sought.

CASE 13-4

INITIAL PRESENTATION

A 42-year-old woman presents to an internal medicine clinic with a chief complaint of intermittent nausea. The patient states that she has suffered nausea for "many years" and does not seem to be getting better or worse. She denies vomiting. She has been to many physicians over the past few years who, according to the patient, have all told her, "It is all in your head." She has no other gastrointestinal (GI) complaints. She has never traveled. She eats a regular diet, and no one with whom she has contact is ill. Upon a full review of systems, the patient relates that she is concerned that she is going crazy sometimes. She states that she is always worried that something bad is going to happen to her, even though she knows there is no reason for believing so. She denies any frank "panic attacks." A chart review indicates that she has been to see seven different physicians in the last 2 years. Despite an extensive laboratory workup, no abnormalities have been found.

PHYSICAL EXAMINATION

The patient is a well-nourished, middle-aged woman who appears anxious and concerned. The remainder of the physical examination is unremarkable.

ASSESSMENT

This case is notably different from the others in this chapter. This patient is complaining of nausea without vomiting or other GI complaints. In addition, her complaints are chronic, appear to be stable, and are not accompanied by any physical examination or laboratory abnormalities other than an anxious mood. The most likely diagnosis, therefore, would be **nausea secondary to a chronic anxiety disorder**. Emotional disturbances very commonly affect the function of the GI tract. In healthy individuals, anxiety occurs normally as a response to stress or life-changing events. Also, stress is a very common response to other emotional disorders as well as medical problems. However, other individuals suffer from primary anxiety disorders, which may be categorized as either panic or general types. Since this patient does not seem to describe panic attacks, a generalized anxiety disorder is more likely. Roughly 5% of Americans may be afflicted, and the number of patients describing anxiety to primary care physicians is undoubtedly higher due to the association between anxiety and other medical illnesses. The diagnosis is confirmed when a patient presents with generalized anxiety or worry for longer than 6 months duration in the absence of any other medical conditions or abnormalities. Internists often encounter patients such as this. The diagnosis may be elusive because it is one of exclusion and because of its variable presentation. Patients may describe a variety of somatic complaints such as difficulty breathing, numbness or tingling, backaches, palpitations, chest pain, dizziness, dysphagia, choking, trembling, and, of course, nausea. In many cases, patients complain specifically of a symptom that relates to the physician's area of expertise. A generalized anxiety disorder may appear almost anytime from childhood to middle age. The exact pathophysiology is as yet uncertain, but most likely involves an imbalance of norepinephrine or serotonin levels in the brain. Fortunately, newer anxiolytic agents such as buspirone have proven effective in the treatment of this disorder. Screening blood tests that must be ordered include a complete blood count (CBC), chemistry panel, and thyroid tests to rule out liver and kidney dysfunction (which may cause nausea, and anemia), and hyperthyroidism (which may cause anxiety). In addition, serious GI problems often result in anemia. If any of these tests are abnormal, further workup is indicated. These tests are inexpensive and, if normal, one may feel comfortable proceeding with a diagnosis of general anxiety disorder. Discuss this diagnosis and treatment plan with the patient and determine whether life-style changes, counseling, or pharmacologic intervention are most appropriate. If the anxiety resolves but the nausea persists, consider referral to a gastroenterologist for possible upper endoscopy.

CASE 13-5

INITIAL PRESENTATION

A 24-year-old married woman comes into your clinic complaining of nausea and vomiting, which began roughly a week and a half ago. She reports that the symptoms are usually worse in the morning. She denies bloody or coffee-grounds–appearing vomit. She also denies fever or other GI complaints. The patient is currently sexually active with her husband and does not use birth control.

PHYSICAL EXAMINATION

The patient is a well-nourished woman who appears healthy and in no current distress. The remainder of the physical examination is unremarkable. A beta human chorionic gonadotropin (HCG) blood test is positive.

ASSESSMENT

The diagnosis is clear in this case, **nausea and vomiting due to pregnancy**. However, it is included here to remind you that pregnancy must always be considered in female patients of childbearing age. In many cases, nausea and vomiting are the initial symptoms, and internists may be the first physicians contacted by patients. Pregnancy must be excluded before other potentially harmful diagnostic tests are ordered. The cause of the nausea and vomiting in pregnancy is unknown but is probably related to the slowing effect of estrogen on the GI tract. Usually, the symptoms are mild and do not require medical intervention. In severe cases, however, patients may become dehydrated and require further intervention. This patient must be referred to an obstetrician for further care.

CASE 13-6

INITIAL PRESENTATION

A 64-year-old man is brought to the emergency room by his wife because he is vomiting blood. The patient has been vomiting up large quantities of bright red blood for the past 2 hours. He had been well up until that point. The patient has never experienced these symptoms before. He denies fever or chills. He has not had any abdominal discomfort lately. His wife reports that he has been a heavy drinker all of his life.

PHYSICAL EXAMINATION

The patient is a thin man who appears older than his stated age. His clothes are covered with bright red blood. The blood pressure is 80/50 mm Hg, and the pulse is 120 beats/min. The heart and lung examinations are unremarkable except for an elevated heart rate. The liver is not palpable on abdominal examination, but the spleen feels enlarged. A caput medusae (plexus of dilated veins surrounding the umbilicus) is noted. The rectal examination reveals internal hemorrhoids and stool, which is guaiac positive.

ASSESSMENT

Without endoscopic evaluation, a definitive diagnosis cannot be made, but this patient is clearly suffering from an **upper GI bleed**. Slow GI bleeds may result in dark-colored vomit that may resemble coffee grounds. In contrast, more massive acute upper GI bleeds tend to produce blood that has not clotted or been altered by gastric juices and is therefore more likely to be bright red and liquid. Bleeding almost anywhere in the upper GI tract can result in vomiting since blood is a GI irritant. This patient's history of excessive alcohol consumption places him at risk for a variety of disorders that could result in hemorrhage from the GI tract. Gastritis and peptic ulcers, for example, are much more common in patients who use large amounts of alcohol. Of primary concern in this patient would be bleeding esophageal varices because bleeding in this area is usually prolonged and can be massive and life-threatening. Cirrhosis of the liver, as a result of alcohol, post-necrosis, or other etiology, causes increased resistance of blood flow through the liver. As a result, the hydrostatic pressure in the portal vein and its branches can also be elevated, hence the name "portal hypertension." Blood from the esophageal veins drains into the left gastric vein and then into the portal vein. If portal hypertension becomes significant enough to result in the dilatation and breakage of one or more of these vessels, then profuse bleeding occurs. In a similar manner, portal hypertension in the splenic vein, periumbilical veins, and the inferior and middle rectal veins may result in splenomegaly, caput medusae, and internal hemorrhoids respectively. This patient shows signs of significant blood loss, hypotension, tachycardia, and signs of portal hypertension. An emergency consultation with a gastroenterologist for an immediate upper endoscopy is necessary. Blood should be drawn for hematocrit, intravenous fluids started, and blood for possible transfusion ordered. If bleeding esophageal varices are found as expected, various modes of medical, surgical, and endoscopic treatment may be considered. The same holds true for actively bleeding gastric or duodenal ulcers.

CASE 13-7

INITIAL PRESENTATION

A 32-year-old man returns to your office complaining of nausea and vomiting. He was last seen in the office 4 days ago for sinusitis. At that time, he was placed on a decongestant and erythromycin. He is allergic to penicillin. At the time of the last visit, the patient complained of headaches and a greenish postnasal discharge as well as congestion and slight stomach upset. Three days ago he began noting waves of more severe nausea and has vomited once. No blood or coffee-grounds material was noted in the vomitus. He reports that the headaches, congestion, and production of mucus have diminished slightly. He denies other symptoms or risk factors.

PHYSICAL EXAMINATION

Generally, the patient is a well-nourished man who appears his stated age and in mild discomfort. HEENT is remarkable for slight tenderness to percussion of the maxillary and frontal sinuses, which is slightly improved from the last visit. Chest and lungs are unremarkable. Abdominal examination shows positive bowel sounds. No organomegaly or masses are noted. The remainder of the physical examination is within normal limits.

ASSESSMENT

Upper respiratory infections commonly cause slight stomach upset due to the irritation of swallowed mucus. Occasionally sinusitis is associated with inner ear disturbance, and this may cause nausea and vertigo. This man does not complain of vertigo, but nausea from swallowed mucus or labyrinthitis is certainly a consideration. A much more likely hypothesis, however, is that the erythromycin is to blame. **Nausea and vomiting due to erythromycin** or antibiotics of any kind are common. The timing of this patient's nausea—immediately following the initiation of antibiotic therapy—makes this etiology particularly likely. It is not necessarily surprising that he is still noting sinusitis symptoms, and this fact certainly may be contributing to his GI symptoms. Sinusitis is often slow to respond to antibiotics because the infection is "walled off" from the immune system and not well vascularized. Many other medications can result in nausea and vomiting either because of stimulation of the chemoreceptor trigger points in the medulla or because of direct irritation of the gastric mucosa. Among the more common offenders are cancer chemotherapeutic agents, digitalis, and opiates. However, an adverse drug reaction should be suspected in any relatively healthy individual who experiences nausea or vomiting soon after starting a medication. In treating sinusitis, the decongestant is the most important therapeutic intervention, so in cases like this, the antibiotic might simply be discontinued. An alternative would be to switch to another type, such as trimethoprim/sulfamethoxazole.

CASE 13-8

INITIAL PRESENTATION

A 54-year-old man presents to an internal medicine clinic with a chief complaint of nausea and headache of 3–4 weeks duration. The nausea has waxed and waned over the last several weeks but seems to be getting worse. He has vomited twice in the last week. No blood was noted in the vomitus. He denies any abdominal pain, and his bowel movements have been normal. The headache is unilateral, fairly constant, slightly worse when bending forward, and new to the patient. His family tells you that he has seemed a bit disoriented and lethargic lately. The patient has been a heavy smoker all of his life and he had a cancerous tumor removed from his left lung 2 years ago.

PHYSICAL EXAMINATION

The patient appears drowsy and in some pain. He is oriented to person, time, and place. Vital signs are normal. Abdominal examination is unremarkable. Neurologic examination is significant for a positive Babinski's sign on the right.

ASSESSMENT

This appears to be a slowly progressing disorder with some associated neurological manifestations. The history of lung cancer is clearly a risk factor for a **metastatic cerebral neoplasm**. In the first part of this chapter we discussed the initiation of vomiting by the vomiting center in the medulla. In addition to chemical stimulants, mechanical stimulation secondary to pressure from a tumor or increased intracranial pressure from a variety of causes can also result in nausea and vomiting. Obviously, we cannot make a definitive diagnosis in this case without imaging; thus, an MRI scan of the head is warranted. If the MRI is positive, the patient should be referred to an oncologist; if negative or suggestive of other neurologic conditions, to a neurologist.

SUMMARY

Next to upper respiratory complaints, nausea and vomiting are the most common complaints encountered by primary care internists. A variety of etiologies and pathologies can result in nausea and vomiting. Most cases either involve the GI tract or the trigger receptors in the CNS. Thus, associated symptoms are extremely important. The presence of neurologic symptoms should arouse suspicion of a CNS etiology, while diarrhea and stomach pain are

more indicative of a GI disorder. Abdominal pain can be diag-
nostically useful if it can be localized, as we saw in the cases of
cholecystitis and hepatitis. A risk factor assessment should always
include a history of travel, known exposures, and alcohol or other
drug or medication use. Chronic versus acute onset of symptoms
may be very helpful in establishing a diagnosis. Acute, sudden-
onset nausea and vomiting are extremely common and often indicative of an infectious or inflammatory process such as gastroenteritis, cholecystitis, or "food intolerance." Slowly progressing
symptoms, on the other hand, may indicate a more degenerative,
chronic disorder such as hepatitis, uremia, or cerebral neoplasm.
Lastly, it is crucial to assess the potential morbidity and mortality
of the patient's condition. Vomiting bright red blood, for example,
can be indicative of an acute, life-threatening condition such as
bleeding esophageal varices. Emesis with the appearance of coffee
grounds is more likely from a slower bleed as may occur in peptic
ulcer disease. Ulcers that erode into a blood vessel may, of course,
cause vigorous bleeding. In addition, other potentially life-
threatening conditions such as acute myocardial infarction, diabetic ketoacidosis, increased intracranial pressure, and intestinal
obstruction may cause nausea and vomiting and must be ruled out
quickly if these are suspected.

CHAPTER 14

Chief Complaint: Fatigue

CASE 14-1

INITIAL PRESENTATION

Ms. M. is a 30-year-old woman who comes to the internal medicine clinic with a chief complaint of increasing fatigue over the last few weeks. She tells the physician that the problem has been getting gradually worse, and she currently has trouble getting through the day. She has a job as a telemarketer and has been warned recently by her boss that she is not productive enough. Prior to her current job, she worked for 9 years as a salesperson in a plant nursery. She says she has never had these symptoms before and has not been using any chemicals at work. She exercises regularly by jogging 2–3 miles a day but has cut down recently because of her fatigue. The patient denies fevers or chills, cold or heat intolerance, menstrual abnormalities, or changes in appetite, bowel habits, or weight. A very careful review of systems reveals that Ms. M. has noted slight tingling in both feet over the last few weeks. She describes it as "minor, more irritating than anything else." Ms. M. denies any other neurologic complaints such as tremors, memory loss, or confusion. She has no symptoms that would suggest ataxia or paresthesia. She has no other medical conditions. When asked about her life style, she reports that she is a "naturalist." She has been a strict vegan for the last 5 years and takes no vitamin supplements. She has taken ginseng to help her fatigue and feels this has been "slightly effective." She takes no other medications on a regular basis. She does not drink alcohol, smoke cigarettes, or use drugs.

> Exposure to environmental factors is always a consideration.

1. What other information do you need before examining this patient?
2. Do you understand exactly what she means when she says she has fatigue?

Discussion

The workup of fatigue may be one of the most difficult problems for an internist for a variety of reasons. First of all, the complaint is often vague. Virtually any medical problem can cause fatigue. In addition, everyone, with or without known medical problems, suffers from occasional fatigue. Yet another problem is the meaning of the word "fatigue." Patients may use this term to describe a number of very different symptoms such as muscular weakness, somnolence, decreased exercise tolerance, malaise, anhedonia, and lack of energy. Historical precision is essential for a proper diagnostic workup.

Upon further questioning, Ms. M. reports no real change in sleep patterns. She tells the physician, "It is not that I am particularly sleepy, I just do not have the energy to do anything. I feel worn out all the time." She has not noted any muscular weakness. She has not been emotionally depressed. Ms. M. states that, otherwise, she feels fine.

PHYSICAL EXAMINATION

During the physical examination, Ms. M. was noted to be a thin young woman in no apparent distress. Her blood pressure was 122/72 mm Hg; her pulse, 104 beats/min; and her respirations, 16 breaths/min. Her temperature was 99°F. Head, ears, eyes, nose, and throat (HEENT) examination revealed a slight pallor of mucous membranes but was otherwise unremarkable. Her neck was supple with no adenopathy. Her chest was clear to percussion and auscultation. Her heart rate was rapid at 104 beats/min but regular. No murmurs or gallops were heard. Radial, pretibial, and dorsalis pedis pulses were all 2+ bilaterally. The abdomen was soft with no tenderness or organomegaly. No clubbing, cyanosis, or edema was noted in the extremities. No rashes or other skin lesions were observed. Mental status was normal. There were no motor or sensory deficits and no tremors. Cerebellar function was normal. Rhomberg's sign was negative. Deep tendon reflexes (DTRs) were normal as was the plantar response.

3. How would you proceed at this point?

Discussion

As we discussed earlier, fatigue can be very difficult to work up because of its vague nature. In this case, however, we do have some significant clues. First, this patient's fatigue can be qualified primarily as a lack of energy. She has no symptoms of insomnia or depression and no evidence of an endocrine imbalance such as heat intolerance, skin changes, weight gain or loss, polyuria or abnormal physical findings of her skin, hair, nails, or neurologic system. The tingling in her feet suggests the possibility of neurologic involvement and may or may not be related to the fatigue. While neurologic studies may eventually be necessary, these investigations are often expensive. A more productive initial approach might be to focus on all of the signs and symptoms and try to find a connection. Her dietary history may be significant. Ms. M. is a vegan, meaning that she eats no meat or animal by-products. Without dietary supplementation, it would certainly be possible that this patient is experiencing a nutritional deficiency of some sort. The physical examination is mostly unremarkable, except for an increased pulse rate and slight pallor of the mucous membranes.

LABORATORY TESTS

An increased pulse rate and slight pallor of the mucous membranes may indicate anemia. A deficiency of circulating red blood cells (RBCs) reduces oxygen delivery to peripheral tissues and thus may cause a lack of energy. Therefore, a complete blood count (CBC) would be a reasonable first test. Despite the lack of symptoms, which might suggest organ failure or a hormonal imbalance, a blood chemistry screen and a serum thyroid-stimulating hormone (TSH) test may also be done at this point. The cost of these tests is minimal, and they can rule out a number of common conditions that may cause fatigue such as renal or hepatic problems, diabetes, and hypothyroidism.

Laboratory Tests	Patient	Normal Values
Hematocrit	28%	35%–45%
Mean corpuscular volume (MCV)	114 fL	80–100 fL
Hypersegmented neutrophils	Present	
Chemistry screen	Normal	
TSH	0.9 μIU/mL	0.4–4.8 μIU/mL

4. How has the laboratory data narrowed your focus?

Discussion

Clearly, the normal chemistry screen and TSH help rule out electrolyte, renal, hepatic, and thyroid disorders. The CBC indicates a macrocytic anemia, which implies a problem in the proliferation or maturation of RBCs. This generally indicates a vitamin B_{12} or a folate deficiency. The functions of these two vitamins are intertwined, and it is difficult to discuss one without the other. Both are single-carbon carriers that are essential for the production of RBCs. There are only two major reactions dependent on vitamin B_{12} in the human body: the production of methionine from homocysteine and the isomerization of succinyl CoA from methylmalonyl CoA. It is the former reaction that is important for the production of RBCs and involves both vitamin B_{12} and folate. Folic acid is converted to tetrahydrofolate via two reactions catalyzed by dihydrofolate reductase. Tetrahydrofolate is the form in which folate carries one-carbon units. Methyltetrahydrofolate can transfer its methyl group to vitamin B_{12}, which can then transfer the methyl group on to homocysteine, thus resulting in methionine production as shown below:

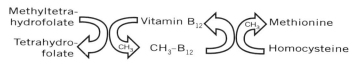

In addition to methyltetrahydrofolate, tetrahydrofolate carries one-carbon units in the form of methylenetetrahydrofolate and formyltetrahydrofolate, which are needed for synthesis of nucleic acids. However, if vitamin B_{12} levels are too low, the above reaction cannot occur. In such cases, folate is "trapped" in the methyl-tetrahydrofolate state, creating a "functional" folate deficiency. Formyl- and methylenetetrahydrofolate levels are reduced, and proper nucleic acid synthesis is impaired. Consequently, a deficiency of either folate or vitamin B_{12} may result in an identical macrocytic anemia.

However, there are some historical clues that differentiate these two disorders. Since only vitamin B_{12} is required for myelin development, folate deficiency does not result in neurologic problems. The exact mechanism of neurologic impairment is still unclear, but probably involves disturbances of fatty acid production and thus myelin production as a result of reduced formation of methylmalonyl CoA (the second reaction involving vitamin B_{12}). This reaction does not involve folate. The neurologic disturbances range from mild tingling in the distal extremities (usually lower) to severe central nervous system (CNS) deformities such as dementia. In milder cases, excessive folate intake may mask the neurologic symptoms as well as the fatigue and malaise. This makes definitive diagnosis imperative prior to treatment because folate supplementation allows the vitamin B_{12} deficiency to progress symptom free until neurologic damage is severe and possibly permanent.

ASSESSMENT

Dietary history may be an important diagnostic aid. Folate is found in green, leafy vegetables such as spinach; folate deficiency is more common in poorly nourished individuals who often have a history of excessive alcohol ingestion. In addition, folate is not stored in large quantities in the liver. Symptoms, therefore, occur quickly following a decreased intake of folate. On the other hand, vitamin B_{12} is abundant in animal by-products. The case presented here is not common. Dietary vitamin B_{12} deficiency only occurs in individuals who do not eat any animal by-products. In addition, vitamin B_{12} is stored in the liver in relatively large quantities; thus symptoms may not occur for several years following decreased ingestion.

Vitamin B_{12} deficiency is more commonly found following gastric or ileal surgery because of the interesting but complex manner in which it is absorbed. Vitamin B_{12}, also called cobalamin, is found in the diet mainly bound to proteins. The low gastric pH, along with pepsin, frees vitamin B_{12} from these proteins. Free vitamin B_{12} is then rapidly bound by a variety of glycoproteins in the saliva and secreted by the gastric mucosa. In the duodenum, pancreatic enzymes once again free vitamin B_{12}, where it can be picked up by intrinsic factor (IF). The B_{12}-IF complexes are resistant to pancreatic enzyme digestion. In addition, this complex is necessary for absorption by the terminal ileum. Virtually any dysfunction along this complex path can interfere with proper absorption of cobalamin. Chronic gastritis or gastric surgery, for example, which may impair secretion of IF, may result in vitamin B_{12} deficiency. In addition, pancreatic insufficiency can result in deficient cobalamin absorption because without pancreatic enzymes vitamin B_{12} remains bound to the binding glycoproteins and cannot be absorbed. Finally, vitamin B_{12} is only absorbed in the terminal ileum and thus resection or bypass of the last 3 feet of the small bowel makes vitamin B_{12} absorption impossible.

We discussed gastritis as a cause of cobalamin deficiency earlier. One particular type of gastritis is due to autoantibodies against parietal cells and is known as atrophic gastritis. This disease regularly causes vitamin B_{12} deficiency, and the hematologic condition is called pernicious anemia. "Pernicious," meaning harmful or destructive, was ascribed to this disorder because of its deleterious progression and the difficulty in diagnosis. The neurologic symptoms are very often unappreciated by physicians until they become severe. Fortunately, the ability to measure antiparietal cell antibodies has improved diagnosis tremendously. In this disorder, parietal cells are destroyed and cannot secrete IF. As a result, vitamin B_{12} must be given parenterally or in very large oral doses. In the case of this patient, however, IF is not the problem. She needs proper nutritional education.

One final comment about the B_{12}-folate relationship: recently, increased blood levels of homocysteine (thought to be an endothelial toxin) have been implicated as a risk factor for heart disease. The biochemical reaction that converts homocysteine to methionine is faciliated by folate, and a deficiency of this vitamin may result in a high blood level of homocysteine. Thus, patients with coronary artery disease may be advised to take supplements of folate. This patient has **anemia compatible with dietary B_{12} deficiency.** Her treatment plan begins with obtaining a serum vitamin B_{12} level. If it is low, the physician will begin vitamin B_{12} replacement and initiate dietary education.

CASE 14-2

INITIAL PRESENTATION

A 44-year-old diabetic woman presents with increasing fatigue of several months duration. She describes her fatigue as a lack of energy and increased somnolence. She denies any muscle weakness or neurologic problems. Her husband reports that she seems slightly depressed. The patient has also noticed a 7–10-lb weight gain during the past several months. She denies any change in appetite and has attributed the weight gain to her lack of energy and relative inactivity. Her husband also tells you that she keeps turning up the heat in their house "to the point where it is unbearable." According to the patient and her chart, her diabetes has been very well controlled for many years.

PHYSICAL EXAMINATION

On physical examination, this woman's vital signs are found to be normal. Her skin is slightly dry, but no rashes or other skin lesions are observed. Her lungs are clear. Her cardiac examination is normal. The abdomen is soft and nontender. The extremities are within normal limits. There are no neurologic disturbances noted except for a slow return on all DTRs bilaterally. Strength is within normal limits. The remainder of the physical examination is within normal limits.

ASSESSMENT

As discussed in many other sections of this book, disease pattern and associated symptoms are often crucial for expedient diagnosis. This case is similar to Case 14-1 in that this patient complains of progressively worsening lack of energy. Without neurologic symptoms or muscular weakness, a neurologic problem is unlikely. The progressively worsening nature of symptoms implies a degenerative process. This patient is suffering from fatigue and weight gain. The other associated symptom, however, is possibly quite significant. This patient's husband reports that she continually turns up the heat. If this is a new occurrence, the patient is noting some degree of cold intolerance. In the absence of fever, cold intolerance suggests hypothyroidism. This diagnosis is further supported by a history of weight gain and the physical examination findings of dry skin and slowly returning DTRs. The concern for hypothyroidism is heightened by the history of diabetes. While diabetes itself can certainly cause a decrease in energy, this patient's diabetes appears well controlled. However, patients with diabetes are at higher risk for thyroid disease, probably because the etiology in both disorders likely has an autoimmune component. Given this patient's findings, we would expect her serum TSH to be high and her serum thyroxine (T_4) to be low. If so, she will need lifelong thyroid hormone replacement therapy. This patient presents a clinical picture of **hypothyroidism.** If the diagnosis is confirmed, her treatment plan consists of oral L-thyroxine with appropriate monitoring of serum TSH.

CASE 14-3

INITIAL PRESENTATION

A 28-year-old man comes to the internal medicine clinic with a chief complaint of fatigue for the past few months. He denies muscular weakness or decreased exercise tolerance. The patient states that he has "no interest in anything anymore." He was recently divorced from his wife for a variety of problems. He is employed as a retail sales clerk but has missed many days of work lately because he has not felt like working. He denies sleep disturbances but states that he often does not feel like getting out of bed all day. On a careful review of systems, the patient describes his mood as "down." He denies any other associated symptoms.

PHYSICAL EXAMINATION

This cooperative man appears his stated age and is alert but somewhat reticent. All vital signs are found to be within normal limits. HEENT examination is unremarkable. Mucous membranes are moist and without pallor. His neck is supple without bruits, adenopathy, thyromegaly, or thyroid nodules. The chest is clear. His heart rate is regular with no murmurs or gallops. The abdomen is soft and nontender with no organomegaly or bruits. No lesions, cyanosis, or edema of the extremities are observed. Mental status is normal. There is no dysfunction of strength or range of motion. Sensation testing is within normal limits. DTRs are all 2+ bilaterally with a normal return. Sensation testing reveals no abnormalities.

ASSESSMENT

This is yet another case of chronic fatigue without evidence of muscular weakness, shortness of breath, neurologic problems, or increased somnolence. Unlike the Cases 14-1 and 14-2, however, this patient's history is largely negative except for a lack of interest in virtually everything and for having social and work-related problems. He has no other physical signs or symptoms. Due to this relative lack of positive findings, social and work problems, and self-described "down" mood, depression is a likely cause of this man's problems. This case, again, illustrates the importance of precise definition of the word "fatigue." Depression is largely a diagnosis of exclusion. As we discussed in the previous cases, thyroid abnormalities and anemias may manifest as fatigue, depression, or both. A screening TSH and CBC can help rule out these abnormalities. This young man is diagnosed with **depression.** His treatment plan includes ordering a screening CBC and serum TSH. If the results are normal, the physician should consider prescribing an antidepressant medication or referring him to a psychiatrist.

CASE 14-4

INITIAL PRESENTATION

A 51-year-old woman comes into the clinic complaining of increasing fatigue. She states that her symptoms began roughly 2 months ago. She has slight shortness of breath on exertion but mainly describes her fatigue as a persistent lack of energy. She denies muscle weakness or increased somnolence. The patient also reports that she has been experiencing hot flashes and increased menstrual bleeding over the past few months. Further questioning reveals that her mother went through menopause at age 49. The patient describes her diet as "well balanced with three meals a day including meat, bread, fruits, vegetables, and dairy." Her weight has been stable.

PHYSICAL EXAMINATION

The physical examination reveals slight pallor of mucous membranes and a slightly rapid pulse but is otherwise unremarkable.

This case bears many similarities to Case 14-1. The patient exhibits progressively worsening fatigue, described as a lack of energy, and has one physical finding (pallor of mucous membranes) suggestive of anemia. There are many different kinds of anemia. Fortunately, history and laboratory evaluation easily differentiate between broad categories, making the diagnosis fairly straightforward in most cases. We saw in Case 14-1 that a vitamin B_{12} or folate deficiency can result in a *macrocytic anemia*. This is because these vitamins are necessary for cellular maturation, and immature cells are relatively large. *Hemolytic anemia*, due to splenic enlargement or autoimmune problems, is caused by destruction of mature and, consequently, normal-sized cells. As a result, anemias of this type are referred to as *normocytic*. *Microcytic anemias* are usually the result of abnormalities of hemoglobin production, as in iron deficiency or one of the thalassemias. While laboratory testing would be necessary for definitive diagnosis, the most likely hypothesis in this case is iron deficiency anemia from excessive uterine bleeding. In Case 14-1, the patient's diet was a major risk factor for macrocytic anemia. In this case, the patient has no immediate dietary concerns but is at risk for microcytic anemia because of her menstrual history. Without iron supplementation, she likely does not have enough iron to maintain the increased RBC production necessary to replace the lost blood.

LABORATORY TESTS

The patient's laboratory test results are listed in the table below.

Laboratory Tests	Patient	Normal Values
Hematocrit	30%	35%–45%
MCV	70 fL	80–100 fL
Serum iron	38 µg/dL	50–170 µg/dL
Total iron-binding capacity (TIBC)	480 µg/dL	250–450 µg/dL
RBCs	Small and hypochromic	. . .

The patient clearly has a microcytic anemia due to iron deficiency. The low MCV reveals small RBCs compatible with an iron deficiency. The low serum iron and the elevated TIBC as a response confirm the diagnosis. (Chronic illness and infection may cause a low serum iron, but the TIBC will not be elevated and the RBCs will not be microcytic and hypochromic.) Once iron deficiency has been confirmed, it is incumbent on the physician to determine the cause. A healthy person loses only a small amount (less than 1 mg) of iron daily, and only a very restricted diet will be inadequate for replacement. A balanced, meat-containing diet provides 10–30 mg of iron a day, but only the amount necessary to maintain iron stores is absorbed. Thus an iron-deficient person can absorb much more iron than one who has adequate iron stores. It follows that most iron deficiency anemias are due to excessive blood loss, and the loss is most commonly from abnormal uterine or gastrointestinal (GI) bleeding. When iron deficiency is diagnosed in someone without obvious excessive blood loss, a thorough examination of the intestinal tract is mandatory unless the patient's clinical condition prohibits such an evaluation. Endoscopic studies of both the upper and lower tract may be necessary to rule out a source of bleeding. Simply replacing iron may mask symptoms until a bleeding lesion has progressed beyond the point where a cure is possible. Cancers of the GI tract are obvious examples.

ASSESSMENT

This patient's history strongly suggests excessive uterine bleeding as the cause, and thus a simple screening for occult fecal blood should be the only additional workup needed. The diagnosis for this woman is **iron deficiency anemia most likely from excessive uterine bleeding.** Her treatment plan includes a referral to a gynecologist for evaluation. Uterine dilatation and curettage will probably be necessary to differentiate between functional perimenopausal bleeding and more serious endometrial pathology such as cancer. In addition, three stool specimens will be obtained for occult blood. If negative, no further GI tract evaluation is necessary. The patient will then begin oral iron supplements. Iron supplementation will continue until the microcytic, hypochromic anemia is reversed and the iron stores are replaced.

CASE 14-5

INITIAL PRESENTATION

A 64-year-old man comes to the clinic complaining of fatigue for 4–5 weeks. Careful questioning reveals that he is experiencing muscular weakness. The patient also complains of intermittent episodes of double vision for roughly 6 weeks. The patient is a carpenter and is having increasing difficulty working a full day both because of visual problems and because of weakness in his forearms and hands. The symptoms are usually quite mild in the morning but worsen throughout the day. Frequent resting helps, but the symptoms become so severe that he is often unable to complete a work day. A careful review of systems reveals that eating has recently become a problem because of difficulty chewing and, occasionally, swallowing. These symptoms also improve with rest.

PHYSICAL EXAMINATION

Neurologic examination reveals bilateral ptosis after sustained elevation of the eyelids. The actions of the trapezius, sternoclei-domastoid, and forearm muscles are all weakened after repetitive movements. Sensory perception is within normal limits. The patient demonstrates no mental status changes. DTRs are normal. There are no other abnormalities on physical examination.

ASSESSMENT

This case is significantly different from the others. The patient is complaining of muscular weakness rather than a lack of energy. In fact, all of this patient's symptoms can be attributed to muscular fatigue. Diplopia and ptosis may be secondary to weakness of the extraocular and lid levator muscles, respectively. Difficulty chewing and swallowing may also be symptoms of weakness of the muscles of the face and the oropharynx. Once it is clear that the patient is describing muscular weakness, the focus can shift to the muscular and neurologic systems. As we have seen before, the pattern of symptoms can be invaluable in determining the next step in patient care. The muscles affected here are primarily those innervated by the cranial nerves. Also, the symptoms worsen with repeated use of the muscles. This pattern of presentation is typical of **myasthenia gravis,** a disease caused by autoantibodies that bind complement to the postsynaptic acetylcholine (ACh) receptors, facilitating their destruction. Acetylcholinesterase (AChE) inhibitors improve symptoms by decreasing the rate of ACh degradation and, consequently, increasing the availability of this neurotransmitter. As a result, AChE inhibitors can be used for both diagnosis and treatment of this disorder. Corticosteroids, immunosuppressive agents, thymectomy, and plasmapheresis have also proven effective for treatment. Other diseases of the neuromuscular system such a Lambert-Eaton syndrome may also result in weakness and muscle fatigue. In Lambert-Eaton syndrome, however, limb girdle muscles are more often affected, and weakness may actually improve with repeated use. From a problem-solving perspective, however, it is not so important to identify the specific disease. The point in this case is to understand the different presentations of "fatigue" and the implications of muscular weakness. The treatment plan is to refer the patient to a neurologist for definitive diagnosis.

CASE 14-6

INITIAL PRESENTATION

A 22-year-old college student comes into the student health center complaining of a 3-month history of fatigue and malaise. The patient describes a lack of energy that waxes and wanes over periods of several days. Currently, the patient has no other symptoms. However, he believes the current symptoms began following "the flu," which consisted of fever, sore throat, and "swollen glands." The patient has no other medical problems and takes no medications. He has no history of depression and specifically denies any current symptoms of depression.

PHYSICAL EXAMINATION

The physical examination is unremarkable except for the patient's affect, which appears somewhat subdued. Initial laboratory testing was done at the time of the patient's original illness. As a result of an error in record keeping, the results were lost until now. The CBC revealed a lymphocytosis with a relative neutropenia. There were also mild elevations in serum levels of aspartate transaminase (AST), alanine aminotransferase (ALT), and gamma-glutamyltransferase (GGT).

ASSESSMENT

Without further laboratory testing, a definitive diagnosis is impossible. However, the signs and symptoms strongly suggest an infectious etiology. First of all, this patient is a young and otherwise healthy individual. Neoplasms, degenerative disorders, autoimmune problems, and other such diseases are relatively uncommon in this population. In addition, the initial presence of fever and probable lymphadenopathy ("swollen glands") are highly suggestive of infection. One of the goals of this book is to facilitate the development of problem-solving skills. One's knowledge base is obviously related to one's efficiency in the diagnostic process. However, in a primary care setting, the ability to evaluate risk factors, associated symptoms, and disease patterns can often lead to a correct diagnosis even without a deep knowledge base, provided one can properly obtain information from the medical literature by using textbooks, on-line searches, and other resources. In this case, the history of chronic fatigue and malaise, pharyngitis, adenopathy, lymphocytosis, and elevated liver enzymes is suspicious for **infectious mononucleosis.** Even without knowledge of Epstein-Barr viral infections, the data collected from the history and physical examination should suggest an infectious etiology, which can then be researched. This case is presented here to illustrate this point and the fact that chronic fatigue may result from some infectious diseases. Other viral infectious, as well as Lyme disease, tuberculosis, fungal infections, and even bacterial nasal and oral infections have all been shown to cause chronic fatigue. The treatment plan involves mononucleosis blood tests and, if positive, patient education regarding expected recovery time. No specific therapy is available.

SUMMARY

Fatigue is one of the most difficult problems for the primary care physician to cost-effectively evaluate. Fatigue is a general term and requires a careful history simply to clarify the actual complaint. In addition, the etiology of fatigue is often elusive because so many different and wide-ranging disorders can produce the symptom. In this chapter alone, we have explored endocrine, psychological, neuromuscular, autoimmune, infectious, and hematologic causes for "fatigue." While the approach to a patient complaining of fatigue may seem overwhelming at first, a precise definition of the complaint and an "inventory" of any associated symptoms will usually point you in the right direction.

Index

NOTE: A "t" after a page number denotes a table.